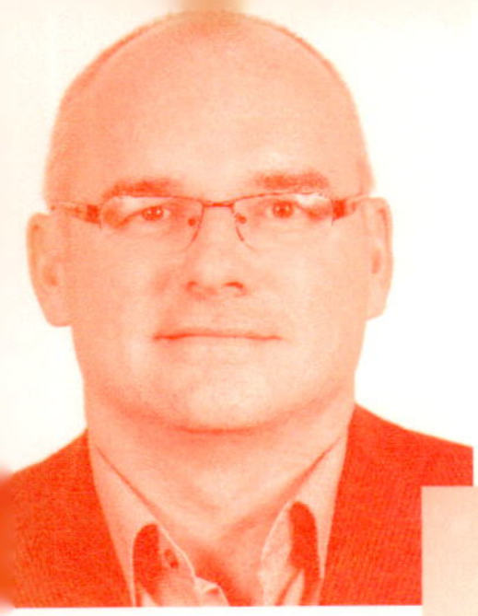
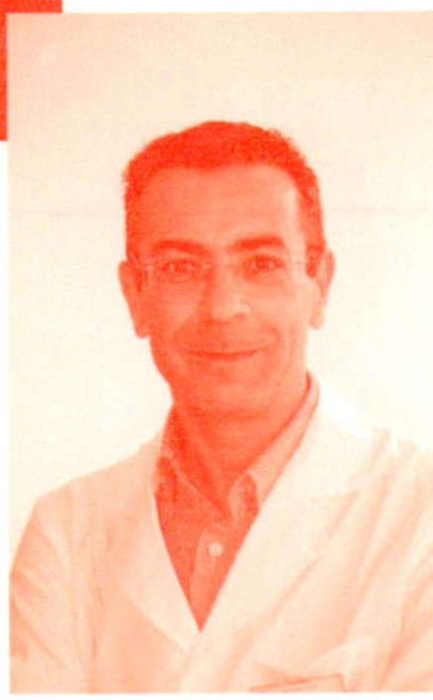
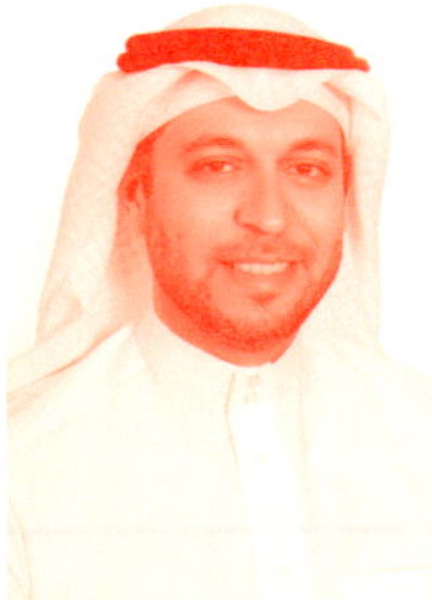
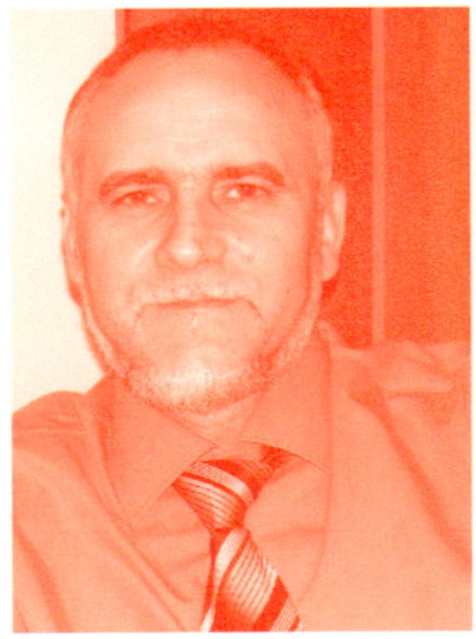
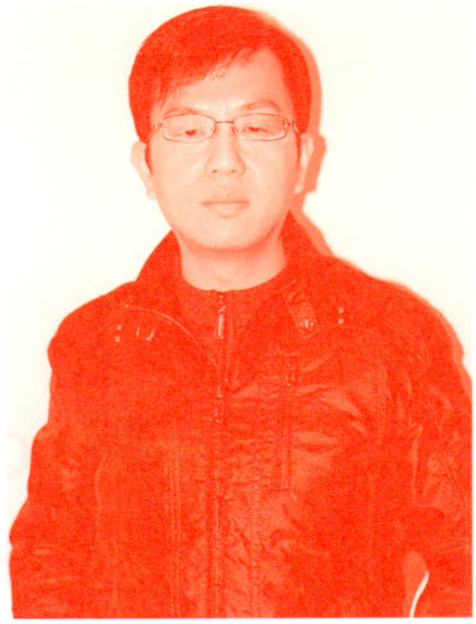
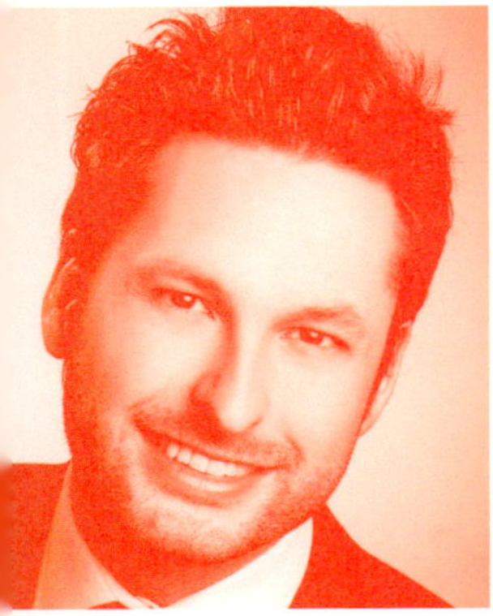
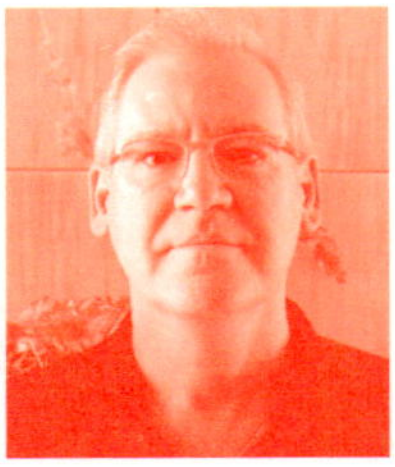

IntechOpen

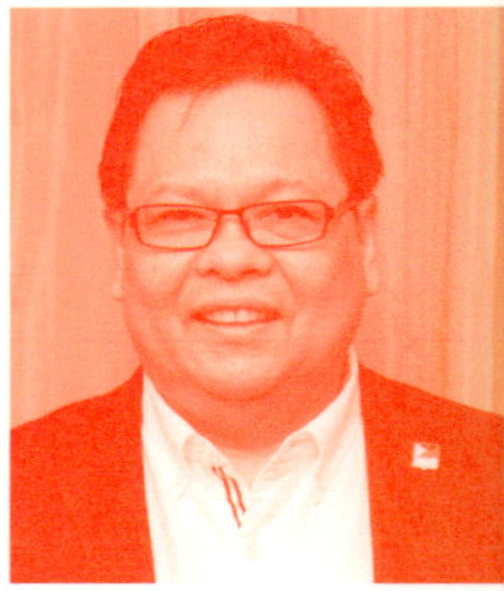
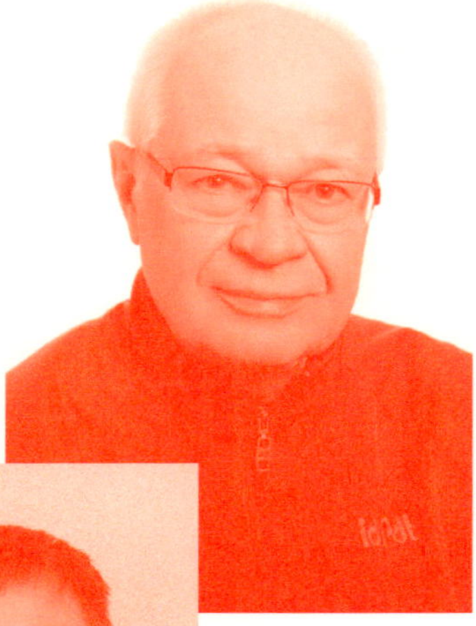
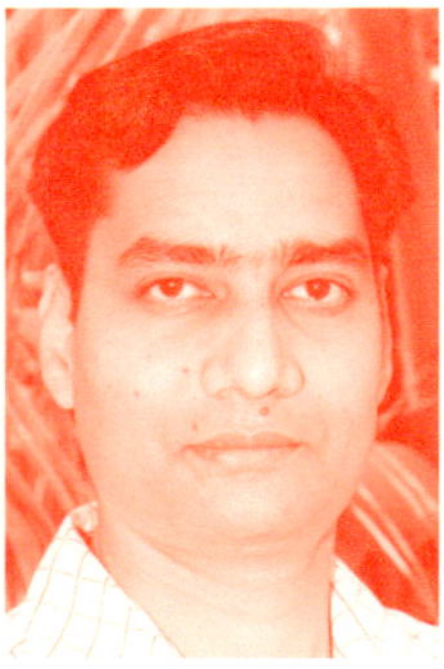
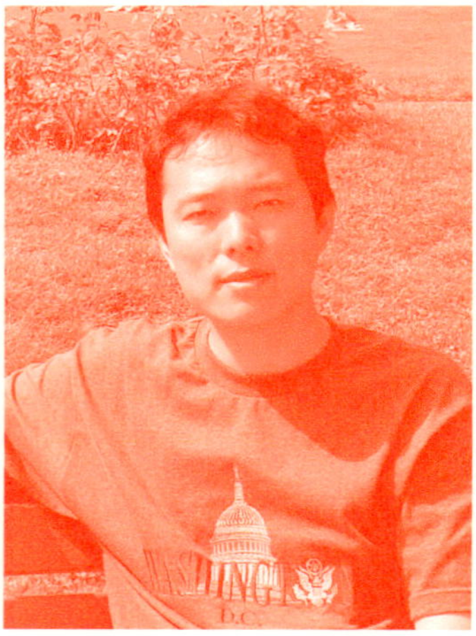
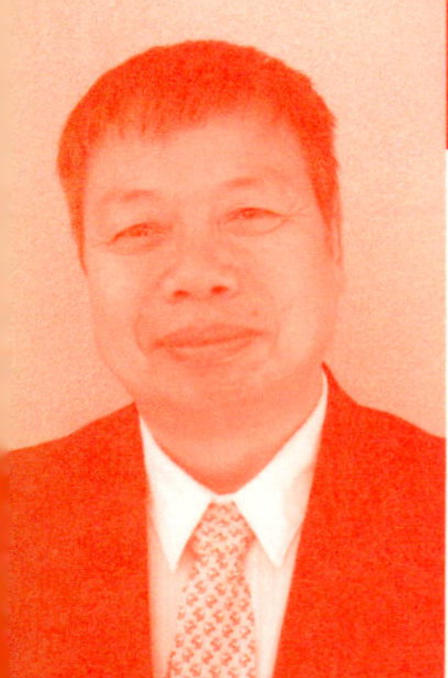
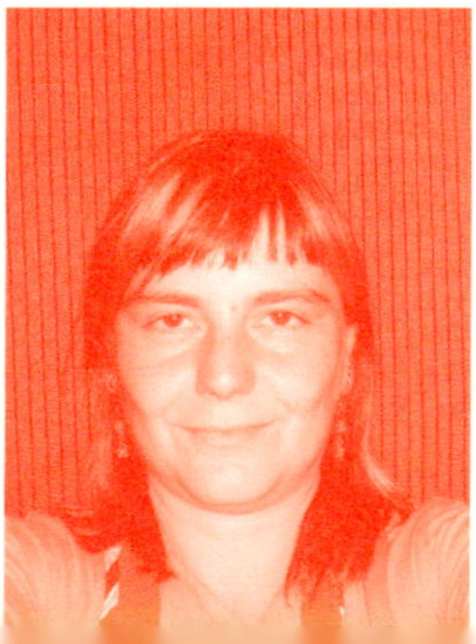

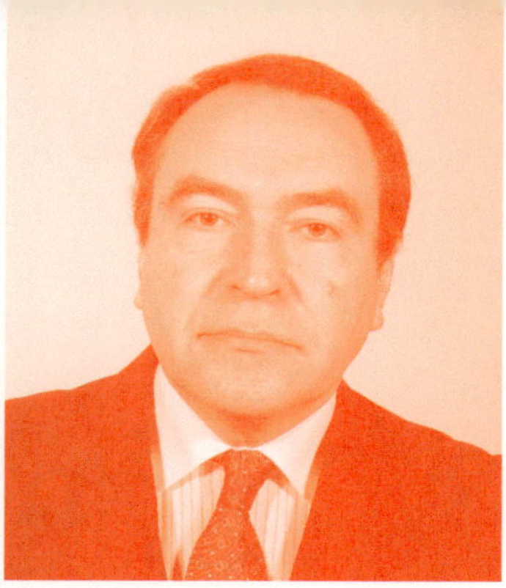
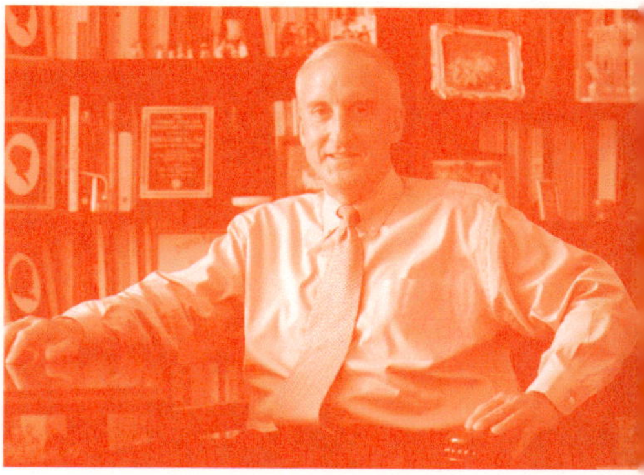
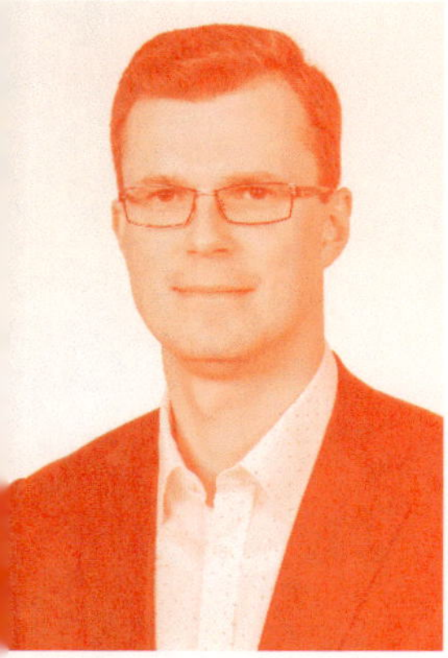
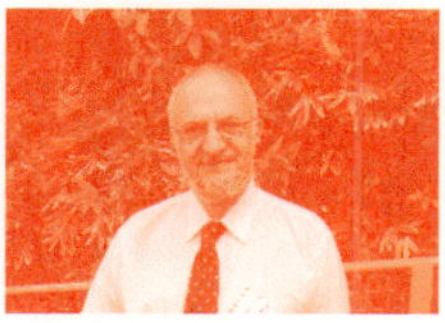
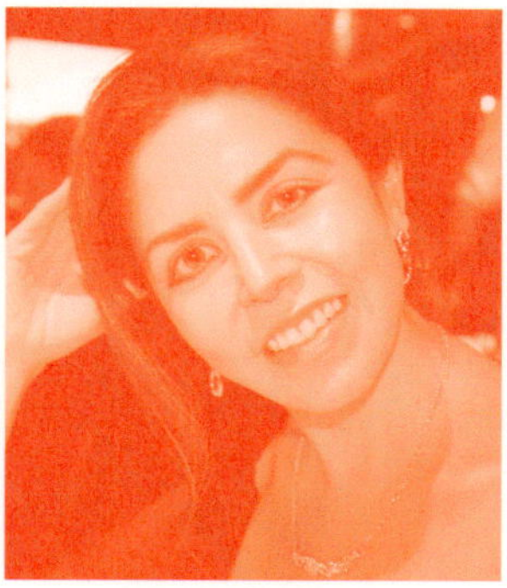

Supporting open minds since 2005

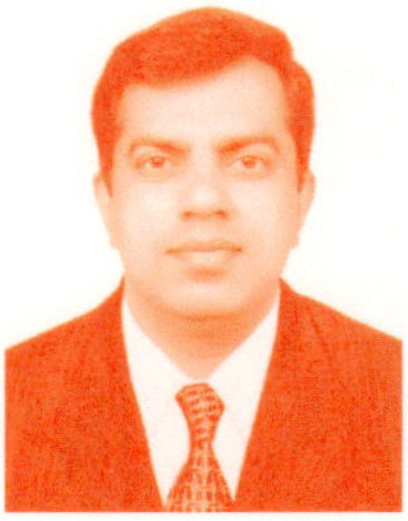
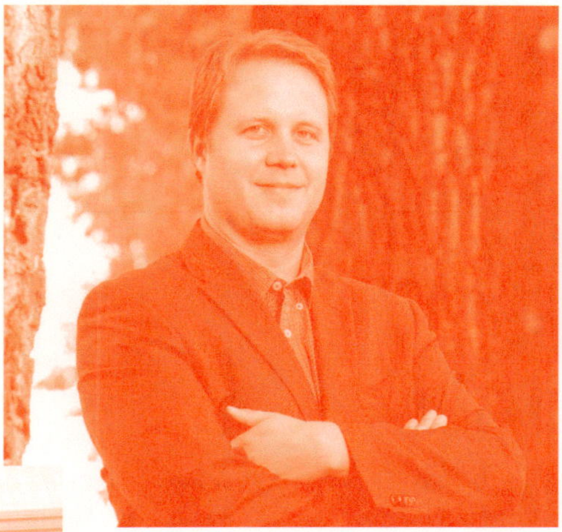
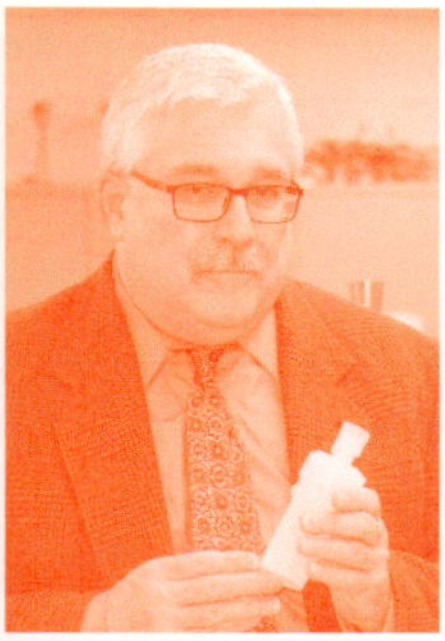
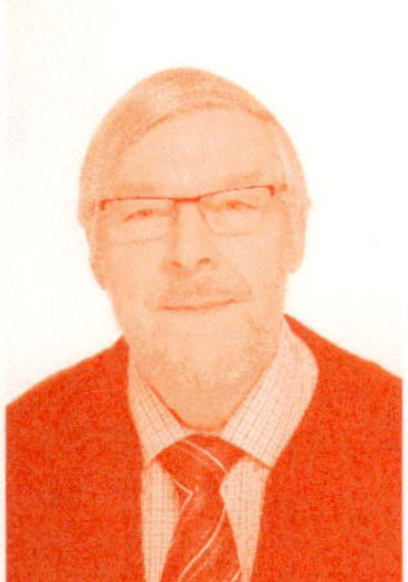
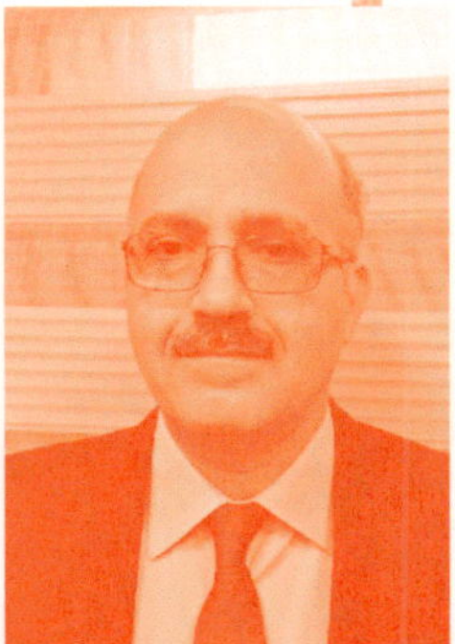
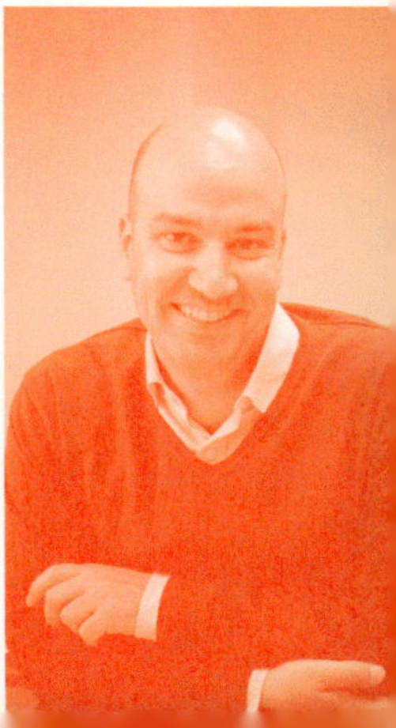
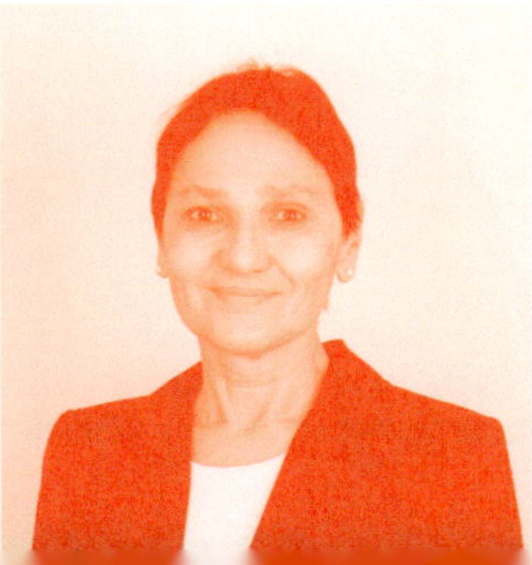

Amyotrophic Lateral Sclerosis - Recent Advances and Therapeutic Challenges
http://dx.doi.org/10.5772/intechopen.78121
Edited by Muralidhar L. Hegde

Contributors
Fatima Pedrosa Domellöf, Luis Bermúdez-Guzmán, Alejandro Leal, Haibo Wang, Muralidhar L. Hegde, Joy Mitra, Arijit Dutta, Patrick Sung, Robert Hromas, David L. Mack, Alec S.T. Smith, Changho Chun, Mark Bothwell, Cristina Cereda, Orietta Pansarasa, Stella Gagliardi, Daisy Sproviero, Ludo Van Den Bosch, Laura Fumagalli, Wenting Guo

First published in London, United Kingdom, 2020 by IntechOpen
IntechOpen is the global imprint of INTECHOPEN LIMITED, registered in England and Wales, registration number: 11086078, 5 Princes Gate Court, London, SW7 2QJ, United Kingdom
Printed in Croatia

British Library Cataloguing-in-Publication Data
A catalogue record for this book is available from the British Library

Additional hard and PDF copies can be obtained from orders@intechopen.com

Amyotrophic Lateral Sclerosis - Recent Advances and Therapeutic Challenges
Edited by Muralidhar L. Hegde
p. cm.
Print ISBN 978-1-83880-580-7
Online ISBN 978-1-83880-581-4
eBook (PDF) ISBN 978-1-83880-582-1

Meet the editor

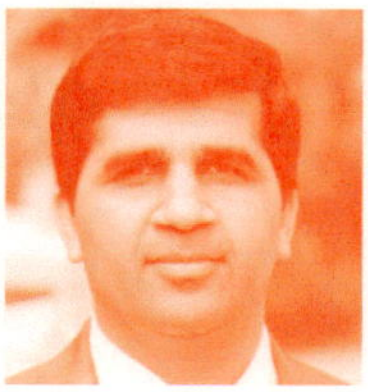

Dr. Hegde is Associate Professor at Houston Methodist Research Institute (HMRI), Houston, Texas, USA. He also holds adjunct faculty appointments at Weill Medical College of Cornell University and Texas A&M University. Dr. Hegde directs a research program focused on delineating the molecular insights into the involvement of genome damage/repair responses in human brain pathologies and developing novel mechanism-based treatment strategies for these diseases. Amyotrophic Lateral Sclerosis is a major focus of Dr. Hegde's research program, with recent publications in prestigious journals that include *Nature Communications*, *PNAS* and *JBC* on this topic. Dr. Hegde's research has been continuously funded by multiple grants from the National Institutes of Health and other foundations. He serves on the editorial boards of half a dozen journals.

Contents

Preface

Despite significant advances in our understanding of the pathological and biochemical changes that are associated with the motor neuron disease Amyotrophic Lateral Sclerosis (ALS), no cure currently exists. Although available treatments can temporarily slow disease progression, they are unable to prevent neuronal death. The groundbreaking discoveries in 2006 that implicated toxicity of the RNA/DNA-binding proteins TDP-43 and FUS in ALS triggered a flurry of research activities towards understanding the neurobiology and pathology of these proteins. Resultantly, the involvement of more than a dozen additional factors (e.g., C9ORF72, profilin, senataxin, etc.) was subsequently reported. Still, how these factors trigger neuronal dysfunction remains unclear, which has been a roadblock in the development of more effective therapeutics. The relative contribution of 'gain-of-toxicity' or 'loss-of-function' of ALS-linked factors is a key question. While initial research focused on RNA processing defects, recent studies demonstrated a widespread imbalance in genome damage versus repair rates, thus opening avenues for potential DNA repair-based therapeutics. This book debates recent advances in our understanding of the ALS group of diseases and outlines future directions for research activities towards finding a cure for these debilitating brain diseases. The diverse but complementary chapters highlight the need for an overarching approach to unravel the fundamental mechanisms of disease initiation and progression that will ultimately allow scientists and clinicians to design effective ways to develop improved treatment protocols for ALS patients.

The book contains eight chapters that cover both basic research/methodologies and therapeutic advances in the area of ALS, with a particular focus on emerging science and concepts. Both common and rare subsets of ALS are covered, including sporadic and inherited disease. Chapters address various topics, such as ALS-associated etiological factors TDP-43, FUS, and senataxin alongside emerging research on genome repair defects, mitochondrial dysfunction, exosomes, non-coding RNA/ biomarker discovery, R-loop as well as the recent advances in ALS therapy and utilization of axonal transport for drug delivery. These chapters are contributed by esteemed scientists from the United States, Italy, Sweden, Belgium and Costa Rica.

The editor would like to express his sincere gratitude to the chapter authors for their invaluable contributions.

Dr. Muralidhar L. Hegde, PhD, FABAP
Department of Neurosurgery,
Center for Neuroregeneration,
Houston Methodist Research Institute,
Affiliate of Weill Medical College,
New York, Houston, Texas, USA

Section 1

New Paradigm of Genome Instability and DNA Repair Defects in ALS

Chapter 1

The Role of TDP-43 in Genome Repair and beyond in Amyotrophic Lateral Sclerosis

Joy Mitra and Muralidhar L. Hegde

Abstract

The pathology of the RNA-/DNA-binding protein TDP-43, first implicated a decade ago in the motor neuron disease amyotrophic lateral sclerosis (ALS), has been subsequently linked to a wide spectrum of neurodegenerative diseases, including frontotemporal dementia (FTD), Alzheimer's disease (AD), and related dementia-associated disorders. ALS, also known as Lou Gehrig's disease, is a progressive, degenerative motor neuron disorder, characterized by a diverse etiopathology. TDP-43 pathology, mediated by a combination of several mutations in the *TARDBP* gene and stress factors, has been linked to more than 97% of ALS patients. We recently identified, for the first time, the critical involvement of TDP-43 in neuronal genome maintenance and the repair of DNA double-strand breaks (DSBs). Our studies showed that TDP-43 regulates the DNA break-sealing activities of the XRCC4-DNA Ligase 4 (LIG4) complex in DSB repair, suggesting that loss of genomic integrity in TDP-43-associated neurodegeneration may be amenable to a DNA repair-based intervention. In this chapter, we discuss the broader aspects of TDP-43 toxicity-induced pathomechanisms, including the emerging role of TDP-43 in neuronal DSB repair and its synergistic genotoxic effects with other neurodegeneration-associated etiologies that contribute significantly to neuronal dysfunction. We also discuss potential future perspectives and underscore how unraveling the molecular basis and implications of TDP-43-induced genome instability in ALS could guide the development of neuroprotective therapies.

Keywords: TDP-43, DNA damage, DNA double-strand breaks, nonhomologous end joining, XRCC4-DNA ligase 4, ALS, stress granule, Rab11, neurodegeneration

1. TDP-43 pathology: a predominant player in ALS

Transactive response DNA-binding protein 43 (TDP-43) is a versatile 43 kDa DNA-/RNA-binding protein of the heterogeneous nuclear ribonucleoprotein (hnRNP) family. TDP-43's cytosolic aggregation and inclusion body formation are the key pathologic hallmarks of amyotrophic lateral sclerosis (ALS) and frontotemporal dementia (FTD) [1–3]. In these progressive motor neuron diseases, TDP-43 pathology manifests as the tau- and synuclein- negative and ubiquitin-positive inclusions in the anterior horn, spinal cord, neocortex, and hippocampus regions of the brain. In the last decade, tremendous scientific investigations have been carried out to understand the etiopathologies of TDP-43 toxicity in ALS and FTD. These studies demonstrated that TDP-43 pathology-linked ALS is one of the most complex neurological diseases due to TDP-43 pathomechanisms overlapping with other ALS-causing genes, such as C9orf72 [4–6], valosin-containing protein (VCP) [7–9], fused in sarcoma (FUS) [10], optineurin (OPTN) [11], ubiquilin 2 (UBQLN2) [12, 13], and ataxin 2 (ATXN2) [14, 15]. Strikingly, TDP-43 pathology has been detected in more than 97% of sporadic ALS cases (>90%), making it a predominant player in most ALS patients.

1.1 Familial and sporadic ALS

Due to highly overlapping symptoms, determining the sporadic or familial nature of the ALS disease at its time of onset is difficult based on clinical features alone. Familial ALS (FALS) is predicted based on genetic screening for *TARDBP* mutation(s) in the patient and matching the same mutation in the family member(s) with a positive clinical/medical history of neurodegeneration and dementia in the juvenile or early stage of life. Race, age, and gender are risk factors for progression of FALS. FALS incidences vary significantly from 5 to 10% among all ALS cases. The disease is more common in Caucasian men and women than African, Asian, and Hispanic populations [16]. Notably, clusters of ALS incidences have been associated with socio-economic conditions along with race. According to Centers for Disease Control and Prevention, ALS prevalence is highest in the Midwest and Northeast of US main land (5.7 and 5.5 per 100,000 population, respectively) [17]. In Europe, the prevalence of FALS was lower in the southern part [18]. Studies show that men are at slightly higher risk than women, with an average age of onset ~60 years. Patients usually survive for 1.5–4 years after diagnosis, depending on the disease aggressiveness [19].

FALS associated pathology affects anterior horn motor neurons in the cervical and lumbosacral regions in the spinal cord, frontal cortex, and cranial nerve motor neurons in the pons and medulla segments of brainstem. Both sporadic ALS (SALS) and FALS pathologies are associated with upper and/or lower motor neurons of the spinal cord. Upper motor neuron diseases accompany degeneration of lateral corticospinal tracts leading to hyperreflexia/spasticity and cardiac arrest. Conversely, lower motor neuron death leads to muscle atrophy and denervation.

FALS cases fall into to three categories, namely, autosomal dominant, autosomal recessive, and X-linked dominant. Autosomal dominance is the most common inherited pattern among the FALS cases, where a mutation in one copy of the ALS-linked gene is sufficient to develop ALS conditions. These patients usually have a strong positive family history and their children bear 50% risk of developing ALS. However, autosomal dominance can also happen in apparently sporadic ALS (because the genetic inheritance is unknown or poor medical history) with de novo dominant mutation(s). In such cases, patients' siblings may have very low risk but children may have up to 50% risk of developing ALS. To date, more than 50 mutations in *TARDBP* gene have been identified in ALS etiopathologies [20]. In addition, a study on a German cohort of non-SOD1 FALS patients revealed mutations in *TARDBP*, suggesting *TARDBP* gene mutation screening should be crucial among non-SOD1 FALS patients [21]. The known *TARDBP* mutations in FALS are G290A, G298S, A315T, M337V, N345K, A382T, and I383V; some of the common mutations identified in SALS are D169G, G287S, G294A, Q331K, G348C, R361S, and N390S/D (**Figure 1**) [21–27]. Most of these *TARDBP* mutations are located within exon 6, as commonly found in Caucasian and European ALS patients; however, a large cohort of Han Chinese population with non-SOD1 SALS did not show any such mutations in exon 6 [28].

SALS has been reported in an increasing number among people exposed to lead or other heavy metals [29–31], smoking [32, 33], and pesticides [34]. Increased exposure to organochlorine pesticides, biphenyls, and brominated flame retardants

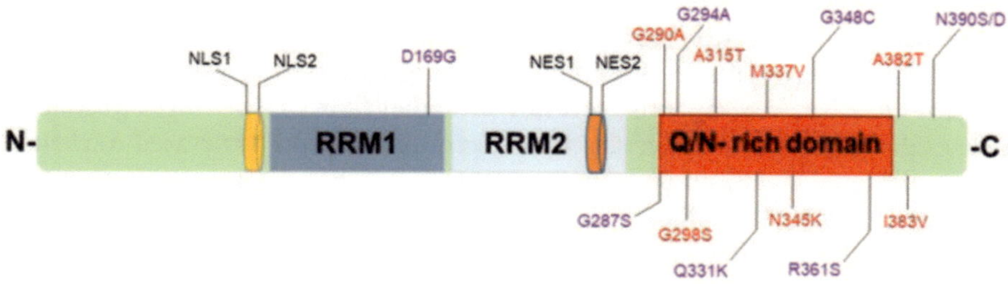

Figure 1.
TDP-43 protein's structural organization. Schematic representation of TDP-43 protein structure shows N-terminal domain of TDP-43 consists of highly ordered nucleic acid binding domains, namely, RNA recognition motifs (RRM) 1 and 2. RRM1 domain follows a bifurcated nuclear localization signal sequence (82–98aa)—NLS1 and NLS2. RRM1 domain spans from 104 to 176aa. RRM2 domain ranges from 192aa to 262aa including bifurcated nuclear export signal sequence (239–250aa)—NES1 and NES2. Later part in the C-terminal domain is mostly disordered and contains majority of the pathogenic mutational hotspots. Familial ALS-related mutations are indicated in red, and sporadic ALS-linked mutations are in blue color.

used in household furniture is associated with higher risk for ALS [35–37]. Interestingly, while smoking has been shown to predispose individuals to ALS risk, alcohol consumption did not show any effect on ALS development [38]. This suggests that diet and exposure to various environmental toxins could increase the ALS susceptibility in the vulnerable population. Most notably, US veterans from the Gulf War [39, 40] and those with head injury [41, 42] are also at a greater risk for developing SALS. By targeted sequencing of exon 6 of *TARDBP* from brain samples of US veterans with SALS, we observed several missense mutations (both reported and novel) and the association of TDP-43 Q331K mutation with DNA DSB repair impairment [22]. Another well-known incidence of sporadic ALS is the Guamanian ALS, which falls on the Parkinsonism-dementia complex spectrum (ALS/PDC). This particular type of ALS in people living in Guam and Rota islands is caused by the consumption of cyanobacteria-infested cycad fruits containing the neurotoxin β-methylamino-L-alanine (BMAA) [43, 44]. BMAA exerts neurotoxicity by incorporating into amino acid sequences and inducing tau pathology, oxidative stress, glutathione depletion, and protein aggregation [45–48]. Genome-wide analyses for ALS-/PDC-associated chromosomal loci revealed three disease-specific loci—two regions on chromosome 12 and the MAPT region on chromosome 17—in these populations [49].

1.2 Unique feature of TDP-43 pathology: dual role of loss of function and gain of toxicity

Given that TDP-43 contains a prion-like domain, its cellular content and distribution are two contributing factors for preventing the protein aggregation leading to the onset of disease. These two conditions are maintained by TDP-43's autoregulatory feedback loop mechanism. TDP-43 is mainly a nuclear protein, but it also shuttles to the cytosol, mitochondria, and other cellular organelles in response to various stimuli. In ALS/FTD pathology, TDP-43 mislocalization, due to pathogenic mutations and/or protein aggregation, is known as the primary culprit for the onset of neurodegeneration. Studies suggest that initiation of caspase-3/7 activation by TDP-43 toxicity facilitates the disease progression by cleaving mislocalized TDP-43 into 35 and 25 kDa fragments. These highly aggregation-prone fragments promote inclusion body formations with the hyperphosphorylated and polyubiquitinated C-terminal domain of TDP-43 [50, 51]. In addition to the C-terminal fragment, full-length and homo-dimerized TDP-43 also has been identified in the spinal cord and brain of ALS patients [52, 53]. Furthermore, recent findings have highlighted that this protein aggregation enhances the aggregation propensities of other prion-like domain containing proteins. The interaction of these prion-like proteins increasing the disease complexity severalfold higher than that of single-protein toxicities [54]. TDP-43's cellular shuttling is regulated by the bifurcated nuclear localization signal (NLS) and nuclear export signal (NES) sequences (**Figure 1**), and loss of either of these signal sequences could be deleterious for cell survival. In vitro studies expressing NLS-deleted TDP-43 found accelerated cytoplasmic aggregate formation along with aberrant RNA processing defects [55, 56]. This phenomenon was further supported by in vivo studies with a transgenic mouse model and transcriptomic analysis in ALS/FTD human brain samples, which revealed significantly altered mRNA splicing of histones and aberrant chromatin remodeling following cytosolic accumulation of toxic TDP-43 [57]. Almost all of the pathogenic sporadic and familial mutations in TDP-43 induce its nuclear clearance and cytosolic sequestration to varying extents. However, in vitro studies with the FALS-linked, NLS-specific A90V mutation in TDP-43 found disease-like detergent insoluble cytosolic aggregates, confirming the crucial role of NLS/NES sequences in TDP-43 homeostasis, and further suggesting cytosolic aggregation of TDP-43 is a determining factor in motor neuron death [58, 59].

Persistent neuroinflammation is considered one of the leading causes for motor neuron death in ALS/FTD and also affects patients' therapeutic response. Innate immune responses, including microglial hyperactivation and astrogliosis, were consistently documented in human postmortem ALS human brain and spinal cord, as well as brains from ALS-model mice [60–63]. TDP-43 plays a vital role in regulation of neuroinflammation by inhibiting NF-κB activation, possibly through competitive binding to importin α3 [64]. TDP-43 depletion or nuclear loss induces extracellular secretion of TNF-α and enhanced nuclear localization of NF-κB p65 in glia and neurons [65–67]. Furthermore, inflammatory responses increase nuclear loss of TDP-43 and progression of ALS/FTD pathology.

2. Broad functions of TDP-43 in central nervous system (CNS)

2.1 RNA transactions

Extensive research in the last decade on TDP-43 toxicity in ALS has established that TDP-43 has multiple functions, including autoregulation of its levels through a negative feedback loop and controlling a diverse set of RNA-associated mechanisms, including pre-mRNA processing and splicing, micro RNA biogenesis, and RNA transport, transcription, and translation. Importantly, TDP-43 also regulates protein levels of critical RNA-binding proteins involved in RNA splicing, including SRSF1, PTB, and hnRNP L [68, 69]. TDP-43's autoregulation is solely controlled by the TDP-43-binding region (TDPBR) domain, which is comprised of several polyadenylation (pA) sites. The silent intron-7 linked to the TDPBR regulates the alternative splicing of pA sites based on the TDP-43 cellular concentration. In the steady state, pA1 allows cytoplasmic shuttling of TDP-43 mRNA for the appropriate amount of protein production. When overexpressed, TDP-43 binds threefold more to TDPBR and increases polymerase II binding at this sequence, which then processes intron-7 to remove the pA1 signal sequence and enforces the use of pA2 and pA4 sites [70]. The use of pA2/A4 sites makes the TDP-43 mRNA partially retained in the nucleus and leads to reduced production of TDP-43 protein in the cell [71]. Moreover, a recent study on TDP-43 autoregulation using the *Drosophila* model has identified human homolog transcription elongation regulator 1 (TCGER1) of

Drosophila protein GC42724 as having a role in TDP-43 mRNA alternative splicing and nucleo-cytoplasmic shuttling. TCGER1 regulates TDP-43 production through its TDPBR region [72].

TDP-43 contains two RNA recognition motifs (RRMs): RRM1 and RRM2 (**Figure 1**). Each RRM contains two highly conserved RNA recognition segments: octameric ribonucleoprotein 1 and hexameric ribonucleoprotein 2 [73]. TDP-43 RRMs bind a minimum of six UG/TG repeats, and its binding affinity increases with increasing numbers of repeats [74]. However, the binding preference is quite different between two motifs; unlike RRM1, RRM2 prefers a short stretch of UG repeats over long repeats ($(UG)_3 > (UG)_6$) [75].

Amino acid sequence analysis reveals a high degree of sequence similarities in the N-terminal domains of TDP-43 among human, mouse, rat, *Drosophila melanogaster*, and *Caenorhabditis elegans*, suggesting that TDP-43's function is crucial in these organisms. The C-terminal region of TDP-43 is predominantly disordered in its native structure, comprising a prion-like domain and several glycine-asparagine rich patches that contribute to the exon-skipping activity of TDP-43 (**Figure 1**). In vivo studies have revealed that TDP-43 regulates its splicing mechanism via its C-terminal glycine-rich domains [76]. A recent study of TDP-43 knockdown in a *Drosophila* model expressing chimeric repressor proteins demonstrated that TDP-43 in motor neurons regulates RNA splicing fidelity through splicing repression [77]. These findings are in agreement with previous studies reporting TDP-43's interaction with more than 6000 mRNAs in the mouse brain and TDP-43 depletion-induced altered splicing of ~900 mRNAs causing neuronal vulnerability (**Figure 2**) [78]. Furthermore, a recent study with ALS-TDP-43 M337V mutant knock-in mouse model has revealed mRNA splicing deregulation as the major pathological hallmark of mutant TDP-43, even in the absence of any noticeable motor deficits [79]. The mammalian TDP-43 primary transcript produces 11 alternatively spliced variants of mRNA, further supporting the functional complexity of TDP-43 [80]. As part of the hnRNP family, TDP-43 has a similar domain organization to hnRNP A1 and A2/B1 [81]. TDP-43's C-terminal domain interacts with a number of hnRNP family proteins, particularly hnRNP A2/B1 and A1, to form the hnRNP rich complex that is crucial for splicing inhibition [82]. HnRNP A1, a 34 kDa protein, is abundant in motor neurons and has been implicated in the pathomechanism of spino-muscular atrophy [83]. Mislocalized TDP-43 modulates the inclusion of exon 7B in the alternatively spliced hnRNP A1 transcript, leading to the production of an isoform with an extended prion-like domain [84–86]. Because TDP-43 and hnRNP A1 interact directly, increasing the aggregation propensity of hnRNP A1 could strongly influence TDP-43's aggregation in a synergistic pattern [87].

In addition to pre-mRNA splicing regulation, the N-terminal domain (NTD) of TDP-43 plays an essential role in protein stabilization and prevention of pathogenic cytoplasmic aggregation. In vitro studies have shown that N-terminal Leu71 and Val72 in the β7 strand region at the interface are crucial for its homodimerization into dimers and/or tetramers in a concentration-dependent manner [88]. Furthermore, single amino acid substitutions at V31R and T32R disrupt TDP-43's splicing activity and induce aggregation. The L28A mutation strongly destabilizes the TDP-43 NTD and promotes its mislocalization, and the L27A mutation increases its monomeric forms [89]. Recent findings by Chen et al. show that the K181E mutation near the TDP-43 RRM1 domain disrupts TDP-43's ability to process mRNA, induces mutant TDP-43 hyperphosphorylation, enhances detergent-resistant aggregation propensity by several fold, and leads to more wild-type TDP-43 in the nuclear and cytoplasmic inclusion bodies [90]. TDP-43 oligomerization has been reported to be the first toxic intermediate in TDP-43 proteinopathies [91]. An RNA-mediated intervention strategy showed inhibition of TDP-43 misfolding in

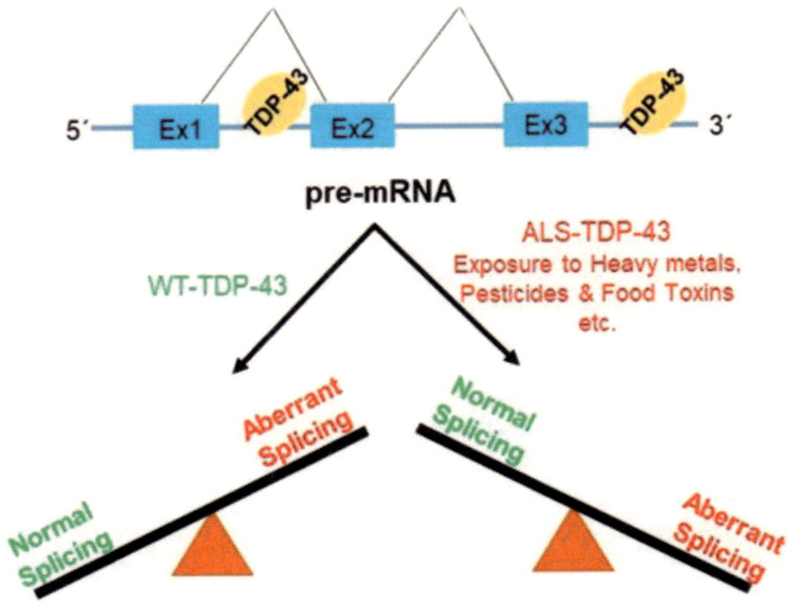

Figure 2.
TDP-43 proteinopathy causes RNA processing defects. TDP-43 being a major functional subunit of spliceosomal complex regulates the RNA maturation processes of hundreds of target genes. Many of which are directly associated with amyotrophic lateral sclerosis (ALS) and FTD. TDP-43, through its RRM domains, binds mainly to intronic and 3′ UTR-located UG-repeat sequences of pre-mRNA to modulate their splicing events. In healthy condition, TDP-43 strongly promotes normal splicing events and inhibits disease-causing aberrant alternative splicing. However, ALS/FTD-TDP-43 pathology induces aberrant splicing several folds higher than normal splicing leading to mRNA dysregulation-associated proteinopathies in motor neurons and glia. Moreover, exposure to various environmental toxins like heavy metals (Lead, iron, zinc), pesticides (organochloride compounds), and food toxins (BMAA) could cause pathogenic alterations in TDP-43 leading to its mislocalization and dysregulation of its splicing activity as a result causing sporadic ALS.

wild-type and pathogenic ALS-TDP-43 mutants, further suggesting a critical role for RRM domains in TDP-43 pathology.

MicroRNAs (miRNAs) are the master regulators of a number of vital cellular mechanisms and diseases, including neurodegeneration and genomic instability. TDP-43 regulates a subset of miRNAs by direct interaction and modulates their biogenesis through Drosha and Dicer complexes [92]. In the brain, neurexin-1 (NRXN1) controls vesicular trafficking between synaptic junctions. TDP-43 has been shown to bind mir-NID1 to suppress NRXN1 expression and thereby inhibit neuronal development and functionality [93]. Given that long noncoding RNA (lncRNA) confers a higher degree of gene expression regulation, TDP-43's increased interaction with two crucial lncRNAs, MALAT1 and NEAT1, possibly modulates the RNA metabolism dysregulation of ALS- and FTD-associated TDP-43 pathology [94, 95]. Furthermore, lncRNA gadd7, which is involved in cell cycle regulation and DDR signaling, orchestrates TDP-43's interaction with CDK6 mRNA that leads to its controlled decay [96].

2.2 Stress granules

Stress granule (SG) assembly is a dynamic, reversible process that promotes cell survival when stress factors are present. Membraneless SG organelles vary in their morphology and building composition in a cell type-specific manner [97, 98]. As long as the assembly/disassembly ratio is maintained in healthy cells, SGs act as the emergency store house for certain classes of RNA and protein molecules to protect them from the various stress stimuli (**Figure 3**). However, altered SG assembly processes are associated with a number of human diseases, including neurodegenerative disorders and dementia [99]. Recent discoveries indicate SGs are critical players in modulating signal circuits determining cell death versus survival in response to stress exposure.

Emerging evidence suggests that TDP-43, but not FUS, regulates SG dynamics and secondary polymerization of TIA-1, which is essential for SG assembly (**Figure 3**) [100]. TIA-1 is an RNA-binding protein and classical SG marker and has more recently been considered as a candidate gene for ALS and ALS/FTD due to its rare heterozygous mutations (P362L and E384K) in the conserved amino acid residues within its low complexity domain [101]. TDP-43 increases its association with TIA-1 in a time-dependent manner in response to the osmotic and oxidative stressor, Sorbitol, in primary glial cells or other stressor-induced SGs in primary cortical neurons and astrocytes [102]. Studies have also shown aging as a crucial modulator of SG dynamics in neurodegenerative conditions. Notably, wild-type and ALS-linked pathogenic TDP-43 mutants show distinct patterns of stress formation rates and morphology. Mutant TDP-43 exhibits faster stress granule incorporation along with rapid increases in granule-size, while wild-type TDP-43 forms increasing numbers of granules with consistent size over time [99]. Apart from the TIA-1 aggregation regulation, TDP-43 also controls the mRNA level of G3BP1, an essential SG initiation factor. The loss of functional TDP-43 or pathogenic TDP-43-mediated G3BP1 mRNA depletion perturbs the interaction between SG components and processing bodies, leading to impaired storage of polyadenylated mRNAs [103]. However, different TDP-43 ALS-mutant variants exhibit differential regulation mechanisms. For instance, TDP-43 D169G does not affect SG formation mechanism, but R361S and A382T variants show loss-of-function phenotypes with

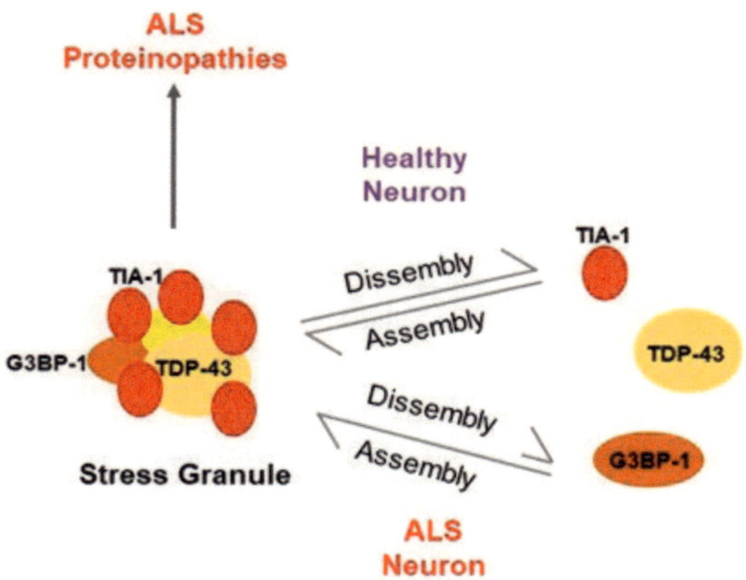

Figure 3.
TDP-43 is a critical component of stress granule. Stress granule formation, in normal condition, is a very important cellular defense mechanism to overcome stress responses. Stress granule assembly and disassembly is a reversible process in healthy cells. It's a membraneless structure consisting of stress granule marker proteins TIA-1, G3BP-1, and TDP-43 as the major structural component. Given that ALS-/FTD-associated TDP-43 pathology induces aberrant cytosolic sequestration of toxic TDP-43, it impairs the reversible nature of stress granule formation mechanism, thereby inducing the seeding mechanism for protein aggregation.

respect to SG dynamics [104, 105]. Interestingly, chronic TDP-43 liquid-liquid phase separation (LLPS) has been observed in neuronal cells and ALS-iPSc-derived motor neurons, even with only a transient stress induction from sonicated amyloid fibrils or arsenite. Early stage LLPS TDP-43 droplets are formed in the nucleus independent of conventional SG mechanisms. Cytosolic TDP-43 droplets formed by transient stress induction gradually incorporate importin-α and Nup62, leading to the mislocalization of nuclear pore complex proteins Nup107, Ran, and RanGap1. This situation inhibits nucleo-cytoplasmic shuttling and clearance of toxic TDP-43 and results in neuronal cell death [106]. Hans et al. have shown that TDP-43 hyper-ubiquitylation-mediated insolubility could happen by multiple distinct mechanisms independent of its translocation to cytosolic SGs [107]. This study shows neither endoplasmic reticulum kinase inhibitors nor translation blockers could prevent TDP-43 ubiquitylation. Moreover, the sorbitol-induced stress response involves impaired TDP-43 splicing activity, whereas sodium arsenite-induced SG formation occurs through oxidative stress, which can be quenched by the treatment with antioxidant like N-acetylcysteine. High-content screening of inhibitors for blocking pathogenic TDP-43 accumulation in SGs from ALS patient-derived iPSc-motor neurons has identified planar aromatic moieties with DNA intercalation properties as the potent small molecule therapy for ALS/FTD-TDP-43 pathology [108]. In this context, it is important to mention that TDP-43 aggregates/inclusions do not completely overlap with TDP-43 associated SGs, rather a subpopulation of those TDP-43 aggregates enter into SGs, and ALS-pathology-linked TDP-43 inclusion bodies are devoid of SGs. Notably, SGs indirectly exhibit positive feedback regulation of TDP-43 aggregation by disrupting HDAC6-mediated pathogenic TDP-43 clearance from ALS neurons and thereby accelerating TDP-43's cytosolic aggregation [109].

2.3 Novel roles of GTPases: Rab11 and RGNEF in neurodegeneration

A common feature in a number of neurodegenerative diseases, including ALS, Alzheimer's, and Parkinson's disease, is the impaired clearance and recycling of damaged and aggregated proteins from cells. Moreover, perturbation of physiological vesicle trafficking systems affects several vital mechanisms in the cells, such as efficient nutrient absorption, failure of cell-to-cell communication, the immune response, and loss of synaptic transmission [110, 111]. Rab-GTPases, first discovered in brain tissue, belong to the major subset of the Ras superfamily [112]. In neurons, Rab-GTPases primarily orchestrate vesicle sorting and trafficking between target membranes through their interactions with effector proteins (coat proteins, kinesins, and dyneins), in addition to tethering and SNARE complexes [113, 114]. Among the Rab-GTPases, Rab11 plays critical roles in trafficking, sorting, and recycling endosomal vesicles around the perinuclear region. Rab11 is transported to the cellular periphery via recycling vesicles traveling along the microtubules and directly regulates vesicular exocytosis at the plasma membrane (**Figure 4**) [115, 116]. Furthermore, Rab11 has been identified as the master regulator for the transport of neurotrophin receptors and β-integrin via axonal junctions in dorsal root ganglion neurons and is critical for their maturation, functionality, and survival [117]. Rab11 participates in different cell survival pathways in neurodegenerative diseases in response prion/prion-like protein toxicity. In the ALS-TDP-43 *Drosophila* model, TDP-43 toxicity reduces levels of the synaptic growth promoting bone morphogenetic protein (BMP) at the neuromuscular junction and increases BMP receptors in recycling endosomes and at the neuromuscular junction. This pathogenic condition leads to larval crawling defects in ALS fruit flies, which are rescued by the overexpression of Rab11 [118]. Schwenk et al. has shown that TDP-43 regulates the number of Rab11-positive recycling endosomes in dendrites (**Figure 4**) [119]. These recycling

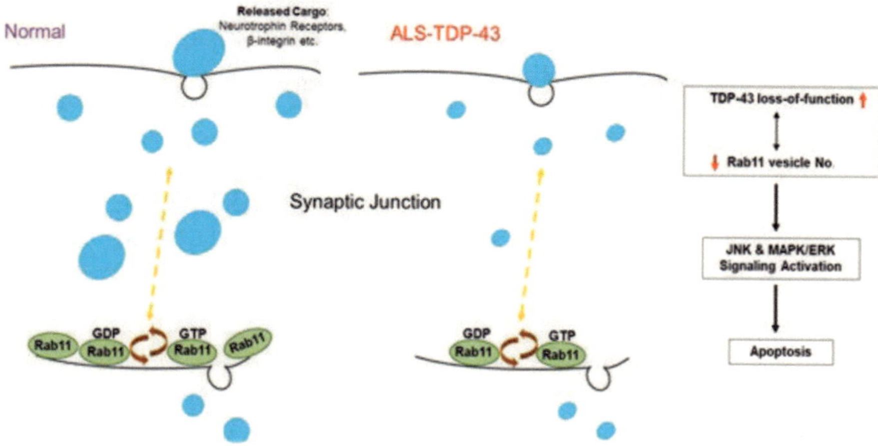

Figure 4.
TDP-43 modulates synaptic vesicle trafficking. Synaptic vesicle trafficking is a crucial mechanism for transporting macromolecules and neurotransmitters across the neuronal axon junctions. Defect in this mechanism may lead to accumulation of toxic waste products in the cells and activation of neurodegenerative conditions. Ras-GTPases like Rab11 plays a critical role in endosomal vesicle trafficking, sorting, and recycling. A study with sporadic ALS patients' brain and spinal cord samples show loss of Rab11 could be closely linked to TDP-43 proteinopathies in ALS and FTD. Loss of Rab11 affects the cargo load capacity and the size of the vesicles as well. This condition in turn activates JNK and MAPK/ERK signaling cascades leading to neuronal apoptosis.

defects in turn affect transferrin recycling in neurons and its decrease in cerebrospinal fluid of patients. In *Drosophila*, a Rab11 mutation induces JNK and MAPK/ERK signaling activation and apoptosis, resulting in defective eye and wing phenotypes [120, 121]. TDP-43 can be phosphorylated at threonine 153 and tyrosine 155 by MEK kinase, a central player in MAPK/ERK signaling pathway, in response to heat shock [122]. However, this unique phospho-TDP-43 variant is not involved in aggregate formation but is instead recruited to nucleoli for processing nucleolar-associated RNA. Further supporting the *Drosophila* model results, we have observed that sporadic ALS-TDP-43 mutations induce the loss of Rab11 in patients' brain and spinal cord compared to age-matched control samples [123]. In contrast to MAPK/ERK and Akt signaling pathways operating in parallel to activate mTORC signaling [124], we have shown that Akt and ERK signaling pathways work in a competitive manner to determine the cell fate. Moreover, in Parkinson's disease, Rab11 co-localizes with toxic α-synuclein inclusion bodies in dopaminergic neurons, and overexpression of Rab11 prevents the affected neurons from degeneration and rescues behavioral deficits [125]. In Huntington's disease, Rab11 overexpression restores synaptic dysfunction and prevents glutamate-induced cell death in neurons [126, 127]. Rab11 has also been found to co-localize with Rab7 and C9orf72 in postmortem ALS brain samples and primary cortical neurons exhibiting C9orf72-induced disrupted vesicular trafficking system in ALS [128]. These findings suggest a broader impact of TDP-43 mutation-induced Rab11 dysfunction on cellular function and survival signaling cascades.

Apart from the Rab-GTPases of Ras superfamily, small RhoA GTPases also regulate broad spectrum of cellular mechanisms including cell-to-cell communication, migration, and proliferation. Given that the mode of GTPase functionality relies on the rate of GTP to GDP turn over and vice versa, dysregulation of guanine nucleotide exchange factor (GNEF) that is responsible for such turnover has been linked to a number of diseases including neurodegeneration. Among this class of proteins with enzymatic activity, Rho GNEF (RGNEF/p190) is directly associated with neurodegenerative disease like ALS, where it not only regulates the function of GTPases for stress survival [129] but also acts as the RNA-binding protein to modulate the stability of the crucial low molecular weight cytoskeleton protein neurofilament's mRNA by binding to its 3′ untranslated region [130]. Emerging studies on GNEF's involvement in ALS has revealed that RGNEF co-exists with TDP-43 and FUS in the neuronal cytoplasmic inclusion bodies in spinal motor neurons indicating a cross talk of protein aggregation and dysregulated cell signaling pathways in the ALS pathogenesis [131]. Micronuclei structures, containing small DNA fragments with clustered DSBs and surrounded by one lipid layer, are a strong hallmark of cellular metabolic stress, exposure to genotoxic agents, and genomic instability leading to apoptosis [132–134]. Notably, micronuclei have been observed in the ALS patient brain and spinal cord tissue samples. Studies have shown that TDP-43 interacts with RGNEF through its leucine-rich domain and forms co-aggregated structures [135]. Taken together, these findings further support the fact that genomic instability is one of the major outcomes in ALS-TDP-43 pathology leading to neuronal death.

3. DNA binding and role in DNA transactions

TDP-43 was first identified and characterized as the transcriptional regulator of HIV-1 gene expression by binding to long terminal repeat TAR DNA motifs [136]. In contrast, a separate study found that when exposed to HIV-1 infection, HIV-1 viral production could occur in T cells and macrophages, even in the absence of TDP-43 protein [137]. As an RNA-/DNA-binding protein, TDP-43 also interacts with specific TG and non-TG repeat containing DNA sequences through its RRM domains, with each domain having specific interaction affinities and DNA conformation requirements [138]. TDP-43 has been found to regulate the cyclin-dependent kinase 6 (CDK6) transcript and protein levels through its binding to the highly conserved long-stretch of GT repeats in CDK6 gene sequence. This binding leads to CDK6 upregulation and thereby increases phosphorylation of retinoblastoma proteins pRb and pRb2/p130 [139]. TDP-43 also acts as the transcriptional repressor and/or insulation regulator for the spatiotemporal regulation of the ACRV1 (SP-10) gene [140, 141]. TDP-43 binds to two GTGTGT motifs in the promoter core region through its N-terminal RRM1 domain during spermatogenesis. In vivo studies reveal that, unlike the wild-type variant, mutations in the GTGTGT motifs in the −186/+28 promoter region leads to premature reporter gene expression in the meiotic spermatocytes [142]. Previously, TDP-43 has been shown to bind both double-stranded DNA as well as single-stranded DNA, with a higher affinity toward single-stranded DNA through binding its RRM1 domain [143, 144]. Qin et al. reported that TDP-43's N-terminal domain is indispensable for its physiological and proteinopathy functions and showed that the N-terminus maintains a highly ordered structure that equilibrates the C-terminal disordered structure by acquiring a novel ubiquitin-like fold that directly binds single-strand DNA [145]. More recently, we also documented in vitro studies on TDP-43's affinity for binding free double-stranded DNA ends, instead of binding a partially or completely blocked terminus [146].

4. TDP-43 in DNA damage response (DDR) and repair

Induction of DNA damage and dysregulated damage response are critical factors for neuronal death in ALS and other neurodegenerative diseases [147, 148]. Studies also suggest endogenous DNA breaks, including DSBs, are routinely generated and repaired in healthy neurons and are essential for the regulation of neuronal gene expression [149, 150]. Besides the transcriptional regulation by RRM domains of TDP-43, no other DNA interactions have been reported for TDP-43. Based on an interactome study targeting TDP-43 in human cells, Freibaum et al. identified the DNA repair protein, Ku70, as one of the interacting partners of TDP-43 [151]. Furthermore, we found that TDP-43's interaction with Ku70 was modulated by DNA damage induction in neuronal cells. Notably, TDP-43 showed pathway-specific roles in DNA DSB repair via direct interaction with the classical nonhomologous end joining (NHEJ) factors XRCC4 and DNA Ligase 4 (LIG4) complex, but not with single-strand break repair factors XRCC1 and DNA Ligase 3 (LIG3) complex. Further experimental studies revealed TDP-43's interaction with a number of NHEJ proteins, including DNA-PKcs, 53BP1, polymerase lambda, XRCC4-like factor (XLF), and the DNA damage response (DDR) factors phosphorylated ATM and histone H2AX (γH2AX). Interestingly, TDP-43 depletion in neurons elicited hyperactivation of DDR signaling without affecting the recruitment of activated DDR proteins to genome damage sites and inhibited the docking, but not assembly, of DNA ligation complex factors (XRCC4, LIG4, and XLF) at the break sites. This suggests that TDP-43 has a crucial role in maintenance of genomic integrity by efficiently completing the rate-limiting DSB sealing step (**Figure 5**). Consistent with these results, neuronal cells with TDP-43 downregulation exhibited delayed DSB repair kinetics and a higher population of apoptotic cells due to the persistent accumulation of unrepaired DSBs than controls. In a correlative study of postmortem human sporadic ALS brain and cervical spinal cord samples, we determined that samples with extensive TDP-43 aggregation and/or fragmentation had greater staining for DSB markers (γH2AX and TUNEL) than their age-matched controls [146].

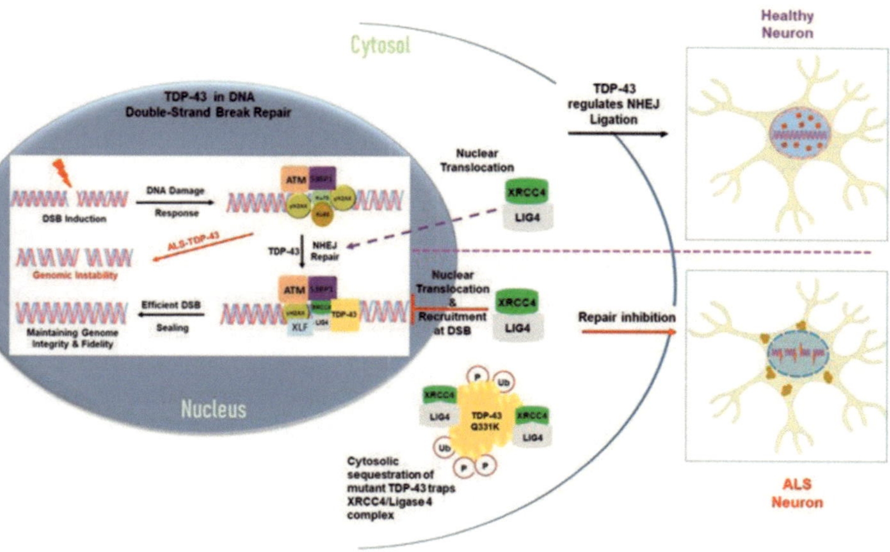

Figure 5.
TDP-43's scaffolding role in NHEJ repair mechanism of nuclear genome. In response to DNA damage induction, TDP-43 gets recruited at the DSB sites and participates in relaying DDR signaling through interaction with p-ATM (Serine1981), p-histone H2AX (Serine139), p-53BP1 (Serine1778), and Ku70/80 heterodimer. More importantly, TDP-43 regulates the most rate-limiting step of the DNA DSB repair pathway—DNA DSB end ligation, through its interaction with DNA ligation complex XRCC4-ligase 4 at the break sites. However, pathogenic mutations in TDP-43 related to ALS and FTD cause enhanced cytosolic mislocalization of TDP-43, thereby inhibiting the DNA damage-induced translocation of XRCC4-ligase 4 complex from cytosol to nucleus. Either of TDP-43 loss-of-function or ligation complex translocation inhibition causes DNA DSB repair impairment leading to nuclear genome instability in ALS/FTD motor neurons.

4.1 Mutant TDP-43 and defective DSB repair in neurons

Efficient sealing of DNA DSBs, which are the most lethal form of DNA damage, is critical for maintaining genome integrity and fidelity. In the majority of the SALS cases, the total amount of TDP-43 does not change significantly, but a significant proportion of the protein mislocalizes to the cytosol and causes ALS/FTD pathophysiology similar to disease-linked mutant TDP-43. We recently linked the TDP-43 Q331K mutation with genome instability and DSB repair defects. In studies with conditionally expressed TDP-43 Q331K mutant, cultured neurons exhibited a strong nuclear clearance phenotype and a higher amount of DNA damage at basal level without the effect of any external DNA damaging agents than control cells. Further investigations showed that TDP-43 Q331K trapped XRCC4 and LIG4 in the cytosol and inhibited their translocation to the nucleus in response to DNA damage induction. These findings suggest that TDP-43 is not only involved in the recruitment of the DNA ligation complex at genomic break sites but also regulates the damage-dependent nuclear translocation of DNA repair proteins (**Figure 5**). These impaired TDP-43 functions in the disease condition leading to genomic instability and neurodegeneration [22].

5. A double whammy of DNA damage induction and defects in their repair in TDP-43-ALS

We and others have observed that the most salient hallmarks of ALS/FTD-TDP-43 pathology, the protein aggregation and inclusion body formation in the cytosol, increase oxidative stress in affected neurons [22, 48, 152, 153]. 4-hydroxynonenal (HNE) increases as an oxidative stress indicator in sporadic ALS patients' brain, spinal cord, and serum. HNE induces oxidative damage to a broad range of cysteine-containing proteins, including TDP-43, through cysteine oxidation. Oxidized TDP-43 mislocalizes from the nucleus to form insoluble cytosolic aggregates in ALS [154]. Such nuclear clearance and cytosolic increase may cause a gain-of-toxicity, leading to aberrant mRNA processing, which in turn exerts a direct DNA destabilization through impaired DSB repair and an indirect repair inhibition by negatively regulating mRNA splicing of DNA repair proteins. Furthermore, the unrepaired DNA DSBs leads to persistent DDR signaling activation through an ATM-mediated signaling cascade that promotes neuroinflammation. This inflammatory response may induce oxidative genome damage and enhanced TDP-43's nuclear clearance, exacerbating the ALS/FTD conditions in a feed forward pattern. Moreover, dysregulation of metal homeostasis has been observed in ALS patients' brain/spinal cord tissues. In the presence of cellular oxidative stress, zinc induces TDP-43's mislocalization and cytoplasmic inclusions [155, 156]. Given that zinc is a crucial metal co-activator for several transcription factors, trapping of zinc in TDP-43 aggregates could globally affect gene activation patterns, including those for DNA repair and response-associated factors, leading to genomic instability.

6. Conclusions: TDP-43-ALS, a case for DNA repair-targeted therapy?

Emerging studies from our laboratory and other groups have shown that in addition to its RNA processing and miRNA biogenesis functions, TDP-43 acts as a key component of the NHEJ pathway for DSB repair in neurons, and its pathological clearance from the nucleus leads to the DSB repair defects seen in ALS and other TDP-43-linked neurodegenerative diseases. These newly discovered paradigms link

TDP-43 pathology to impaired DNA repair and suggest potential avenues for DNA repair-targeted therapies for TDP-43-ALS and related motor neuron diseases. Future studies should focus on a comprehensive delineation of the molecular mechanisms involved in order to develop efficiently targeted interventions. In addition, the implications of these defects in neuronal and glial functions in the CNS of TDP-43-ALS patients and the role of TDP-43 in maintaining genome integrity in non-neuronal brain cells, including glia and astrocytes, are important lines of investigation. By comparing the DNA repair role of TDP-43 in post-mitotic vs. cycling cells, we could learn important mechanistic insights on the selective vulnerability of neurons in ALS.

Recently, an increasing number of studies have demonstrated the role of RNA/DNA-binding proteins in DNA repair. We previously documented the involvement of hnRNP-U, a member of the hnRNP family, in oxidative damage repair in the human genome and its role as a molecular switch between DSB repair and oxidative damage repair when these complex damages occur in a clustered fashion [157, 158]. We also discovered that another RNA-/DNA-binding protein, fused in sarcoma/translocated in liposarcoma (FUS/TLS), linked to the ALS-FUS subtype, participates in break sealing during DNA SSB repair [10]. Because both TDP-43 and FUS influence the final DNA break/sealing step of repair, further investigations in DNA repair mechanisms are critical to developing clinically effective strategies for ameliorating the genome instability of ALS-TDP-43.

Acknowledgements

Research in Hegde laboratory is supported by grants from the National Institute of Neurological Disorders and Stroke (NINDS) and National Institute of Aging (NIA) of the National Institute of Health (NIH) under the award numbers R01NS088645, RF1NS112719, and R03AG064266 and the Houston Methodist Research Institute funds. The content is solely the responsibility of the authors and does not necessarily represent the official views of the funding agencies. The authors thank members of the Hegde Laboratory—Haibo Wang, Manohar Kodavati, Pavana Hegde, Velmarini Vasquez, and Erika Guerrero for assistance.

Author details

Joy Mitra[1*] and Muralidhar L. Hegde[1,2*]

1 Department of Neurosurgery, Center for Neuroregeneration, Houston Methodist Research Institute, Houston, Texas, USA

2 Weill Medical College of Cornell University, New York, USA

*Address all correspondence to: jmitra@houstonmethodist.org and mlhegde@houstonmethodist.org

References

[1] Neumann M et al. Ubiquitinated TDP-43 in frontotemporal lobar degeneration and amyotrophic lateral sclerosis. Science. 2006;**314**(5796):130-133

[2] Arai T et al. TDP-43 is a component of ubiquitin-positive tau-negative inclusions in frontotemporal lobar degeneration and amyotrophic lateral sclerosis. Biochemical and Biophysical Research Communications. 2006;**351**(3):602-611

[3] Maekawa S et al. TDP-43 is consistently co-localized with ubiquitinated inclusions in sporadic and Guam amyotrophic lateral sclerosis but not in familial amyotrophic lateral sclerosis with and without SOD1 mutations. Neuropathology. 2009;**29**(6):672-683

[4] Al-Sarraj S et al. p62 positive, TDP-43 negative, neuronal cytoplasmic and intranuclear inclusions in the cerebellum and hippocampus define the pathology of C9orf72-linked FTLD and MND/ALS. Acta Neuropathologica. 2011;**122**(6):691-702

[5] DeJesus-Hernandez M et al. Expanded GGGGCC hexanucleotide repeat in noncoding region of C9ORF72 causes chromosome 9p-linked FTD and ALS. Neuron. 2011;**72**(2):245-256

[6] Chew J et al. Neurodegeneration. C9ORF72 repeat expansions in mice cause TDP-43 pathology, neuronal loss, and behavioral deficits. Science. 2015;**348**(6239):1151-1154

[7] Gitcho MA et al. VCP mutations causing frontotemporal lobar degeneration disrupt localization of TDP-43 and induce cell death. The Journal of Biological Chemistry. 2009;**284**(18):12384-12398

[8] Liu G et al. Cdc48/VCP and endocytosis regulate TDP-43 and FUS toxicity and turnover. Molecular and Cellular Biology. 2020:**40**(4):e00256-19

[9] Neumann M et al. TDP-43 in the ubiquitin pathology of frontotemporal dementia with VCP gene mutations. Journal of Neuropathology and Experimental Neurology. 2007;**66**(2):152-157

[10] Wang H et al. Mutant FUS causes DNA ligation defects to inhibit oxidative damage repair in amyotrophic lateral sclerosis. Nature Communications. 2018;**9**(1):3683

[11] Hortobagyi T et al. Optineurin inclusions occur in a minority of TDP-43 positive ALS and FTLD-TDP cases and are rarely observed in other neurodegenerative disorders. Acta Neuropathologica. 2011;**121**(4):519-527

[12] Deng HX et al. Mutations in UBQLN2 cause dominant X-linked juvenile and adult-onset ALS and ALS/dementia. Nature. 2011;**477**(7363):211-215

[13] Williams KL et al. UBQLN2/ubiquilin 2 mutation and pathology in familial amyotrophic lateral sclerosis. Neurobiology of Aging. 2012;**33**(10):2527.e3-2527.10

[14] Elden AC et al. Ataxin-2 intermediate-length polyglutamine expansions are associated with increased risk for ALS. Nature. 2010;**466**(7310):1069-1075

[15] Farg MA et al. Ataxin-2 interacts with FUS and intermediate-length polyglutamine expansions enhance FUS-related pathology in amyotrophic lateral sclerosis. Human Molecular Genetics. 2013;**22**(4):717-728

[16] Henry KA et al. Geographic variation of amyotrophic lateral sclerosis incidence in New Jersey,

2009-2011. American Journal of Epidemiology. 2015;**182**(6):512-519

[17] Mehta P et al. Prevalence of amyotrophic lateral sclerosis - United States, 2015. MMWR. Morbidity and Mortality Weekly Report. 2018;**67**(46):1285-1289

[18] Byrne S et al. Rate of familial amyotrophic lateral sclerosis: A systematic review and meta-analysis. Journal of Neurology, Neurosurgery, and Psychiatry. 2011;**82**(6):623-627

[19] Chio A et al. Prognostic factors in ALS: A critical review. Amyotrophic Lateral Sclerosis. 2009;**10**(5-6):310-323

[20] Buratti E. Functional significance of TDP-43 mutations in disease. Advances in Genetics. 2015;**91**:1-53

[21] Kuhnlein P et al. Two German kindreds with familial amyotrophic lateral sclerosis due to TARDBP mutations. Archives of Neurology. 2008;**65**(9):1185-1189

[22] Guerrero EN et al. Amyotrophic lateral sclerosis-associated TDP-43 mutation Q331K prevents nuclear translocation of XRCC4-DNA ligase 4 complex and is linked to genome damage-mediated neuronal apoptosis. Human Molecular Genetics. 2019;**28**(5):2459-2476

[23] Rutherford NJ et al. Novel mutations in TARDBP (TDP-43) in patients with familial amyotrophic lateral sclerosis. PLoS Genetics. 2008;**4**(9):e1000193

[24] Gitcho MA et al. TDP-43 A315T mutation in familial motor neuron disease. Annals of Neurology. 2008;**63**(4):535-538

[25] Sreedharan J et al. TDP-43 mutations in familial and sporadic amyotrophic lateral sclerosis. Science. 2008;**319**(5870):1668-1672

[26] Van Deerlin VM et al. TARDBP mutations in amyotrophic lateral sclerosis with TDP-43 neuropathology: A genetic and histopathological analysis. Lancet Neurology. 2008;**7**(5):409-416

[27] Kabashi E et al. TARDBP mutations in individuals with sporadic and familial amyotrophic lateral sclerosis. Nature Genetics. 2008;**40**(5):572-574

[28] Ye CH et al. Absence of mutations in exon 6 of the TARDBP gene in 207 Chinese patients with sporadic amyotrohic lateral sclerosis. PLoS One. 2013;**8**(7):e68106

[29] Fang F et al. Association between blood lead and the risk of amyotrophic lateral sclerosis. American Journal of Epidemiology. 2010;**171**(10):1126-1133

[30] Campbell AM, Williams ER, Barltrop D. Motor neurone disease and exposure to lead. Journal of Neurology, Neurosurgery, and Psychiatry. 1970;**33**(6):877-885

[31] Gresham LS et al. Amyotrophic lateral sclerosis and occupational heavy metal exposure: A case-control study. Neuroepidemiology. 1986;**5**(1):29-38

[32] Wang H et al. Smoking and risk of amyotrophic lateral sclerosis: A pooled analysis of 5 prospective cohorts. Archives of Neurology. 2011;**68**(2):207-213

[33] Gallo V et al. Smoking and risk for amyotrophic lateral sclerosis: Analysis of the EPIC cohort. Annals of Neurology. 2009;**65**(4):378-385

[34] Bonvicini F et al. Exposure to pesticides and risk of amyotrophic lateral sclerosis: A population-based case-control study. Annali dell'Istituto Superiore di Sanità. 2010;**46**(3):284-287

[35] Su FC et al. Association of environmental toxins with amyotrophic lateral sclerosis. JAMA Neurology. 2016;**73**(7):803-811

[36] Malek AM et al. Exposure to hazardous air pollutants and the risk of amyotrophic lateral sclerosis. Environmental Pollution. 2015;**197**:181-186

[37] Yu Y et al. Environmental risk factors and amyotrophic lateral sclerosis (ALS): A case-control study of ALS in Michigan. PLoS One. 2014;**9**(6):e101186

[38] de Jong SW et al. Smoking, alcohol consumption, and the risk of amyotrophic lateral sclerosis: A population-based study. American Journal of Epidemiology. 2012;**176**(3):233-239

[39] Haley RW. Excess incidence of ALS in young gulf war veterans. Neurology. 2003;**61**(6):750-756

[40] Weisskopf MG et al. Prospective study of military service and mortality from ALS. Neurology. 2005;**64**(1):32-37

[41] Chen H et al. Head injury and amyotrophic lateral sclerosis. American Journal of Epidemiology. 2007;**166**(7):810-816

[42] Schmidt S et al. Association of ALS with head injury, cigarette smoking and APOE genotypes. Journal of the Neurological Sciences. 2010;**291**(1-2):22-29

[43] Cox PA, Sacks OW. Cycad neurotoxins, consumption of flying foxes, and ALS-PDC disease in Guam. Neurology. 2002;**58**(6):956-959

[44] Garruto RM, Gajdusek C, Chen KM. Amyotrophic lateral sclerosis among Chamorro migrants from Guam. Annals of Neurology. 1980;**8**(6):612-619

[45] Arif M et al. Tau pathology involves protein phosphatase 2A in parkinsonism-dementia of Guam. Proceedings of the National Academy of Sciences of the United States of America. 2014;**111**(3):1144-1149

[46] Weiss JH, Koh JY, Choi DW. Neurotoxicity of beta-N-methylamino-L-alanine (BMAA) and beta-N-oxalylamino-L-alanine (BOAA) on cultured cortical neurons. Brain Research. 1989;**497**(1):64-71

[47] Yin HZ et al. Intrathecal infusion of BMAA induces selective motor neuron damage and astrogliosis in the ventral horn of the spinal cord. Experimental Neurology. 2014;**261**:1-9

[48] Guerrero EN et al. TDP-43/FUS in motor neuron disease: Complexity and challenges. Progress in Neurobiology. 2016;**145-146**:78-97

[49] Sieh W et al. Identification of novel susceptibility loci for Guam neurodegenerative disease: Challenges of genome scans in genetic isolates. Human Molecular Genetics. 2009;**18**(19):3725-3738

[50] Li Q et al. The cleavage pattern of TDP-43 determines its rate of clearance and cytotoxicity. Nature Communications. 2015;**6**:6183

[51] Asakawa K, Handa H, Kawakami K. Optogenetic modulation of TDP-43 oligomerization accelerates ALS-related pathologies in the spinal motor neurons. Nature Communications. 2020;**11**(1):1004

[52] Zhang YJ et al. Aberrant cleavage of TDP-43 enhances aggregation and cellular toxicity. Proceedings of the National Academy of Sciences of the United States of America. 2009;**106**(18):7607-7612

[53] Shiina Y et al. TDP-43 dimerizes in human cells in culture. Cellular and Molecular Neurobiology. 2010;**30**(4):641-652

[54] Hergesheimer RC et al. The debated toxic role of aggregated TDP-43 in amyotrophic lateral

sclerosis: A resolution in sight? Brain. 2019;**142**(5):1176-1194

[55] Winton MJ et al. Disturbance of nuclear and cytoplasmic TAR DNA-binding protein (TDP-43) induces disease-like redistribution, sequestration, and aggregate formation. The Journal of Biological Chemistry. 2008;**283**(19):13302-13309

[56] Shodai A et al. Conserved acidic amino acid residues in a second RNA recognition motif regulate assembly and function of TDP-43. PLoS One. 2012;**7**(12):e52776

[57] Amlie-Wolf A et al. Transcriptomic changes due to cytoplasmic TDP-43 expression reveal Dysregulation of histone transcripts and nuclear chromatin. PLoS One. 2015;**10**(10):e0141836

[58] Winton MJ et al. A90V TDP-43 variant results in the aberrant localization of TDP-43 in vitro. FEBS Letters. 2008;**582**(15):2252-2256

[59] Barmada SJ et al. Cytoplasmic mislocalization of TDP-43 is toxic to neurons and enhanced by a mutation associated with familial amyotrophic lateral sclerosis. The Journal of Neuroscience. 2010;**30**(2):639-649

[60] Jara JH et al. Evidence for an early innate immune response in the motor cortex of ALS. Journal of Neuroinflammation. 2017;**14**(1):129

[61] Jara JH et al. MCP1-CCR2 and neuroinflammation in the ALS motor cortex with TDP-43 pathology. Journal of Neuroinflammation. 2019;**16**(1):196

[62] Beers DR et al. Neuroinflammation modulates distinct regional and temporal clinical responses in ALS mice. Brain, Behavior, and Immunity. 2011;**25**(5):1025-1035

[63] Puentes F et al. Non-neuronal cells in ALS: Role of glial, immune cells and blood-CNS barriers. Brain Pathology. 2016;**26**(2):248-257

[64] Zhu J, Cynader MS, Jia W. TDP-43 inhibits NF-kappaB activity by blocking p65 nuclear translocation. PLoS One. 2015;**10**(11):e0142296

[65] Frakes AE et al. Microglia induce motor neuron death via the classical NF-kappaB pathway in amyotrophic lateral sclerosis. Neuron. 2014;**81**(5):1009-1023

[66] Correia AS et al. Inflammation induces TDP-43 Mislocalization and aggregation. PLoS One. 2015;**10**(10):e0140248

[67] Swarup V et al. Deregulation of TDP-43 in amyotrophic lateral sclerosis triggers nuclear factor kappaB-mediated pathogenic pathways. The Journal of Experimental Medicine. 2011;**208**(12):2429-2447

[68] Buratti E, Baralle FE. Multiple roles of TDP-43 in gene expression, splicing regulation, and human disease. Frontiers in Bioscience. 2008;**13**:867-878

[69] Buratti E, Baralle FE. TDP-43: Gumming up neurons through protein-protein and protein-RNA interactions. Trends in Biochemical Sciences. 2012;**37**(6):237-247

[70] Avendano-Vazquez SE et al. Autoregulation of TDP-43 mRNA levels involves interplay between transcription, splicing, and alternative polyA site selection. Genes & Development. 2012;**26**(15):1679-1684

[71] Bembich S et al. Predominance of spliceosomal complex formation over polyadenylation site selection in TDP-43 autoregulation. Nucleic Acids Research. 2014;**42**(5):3362-3371

[72] Pons M et al. Identification of TCERG1 as a new genetic modulator of TDP-43 production in drosophila. Acta

Neuropathologica Communications. 2018;**6**(1):138

[73] Maris C, Dominguez C, Allain FH. The RNA recognition motif, a plastic RNA-binding platform to regulate post-transcriptional gene expression. The FEBS Journal. 2005;**272**(9):2118-2131

[74] Buratti E, Baralle FE. Characterization and functional implications of the RNA binding properties of nuclear factor TDP-43, a novel splicing regulator of CFTR exon 9. The Journal of Biological Chemistry. 2001;**276**(39):36337-36343

[75] Kuo PH et al. Structural insights into TDP-43 in nucleic-acid binding and domain interactions. Nucleic Acids Research. 2009;**37**(6):1799-1808

[76] Ayala YM et al. Human, drosophila, and C.elegans TDP43: Nucleic acid binding properties and splicing regulatory function. Journal of Molecular Biology. 2005;**348**(3):575-588

[77] Donde A et al. Splicing repression is a major function of TDP-43 in motor neurons. Acta Neuropathologica. 2019;**138**(5):813-826

[78] Polymenidou M et al. Long pre-mRNA depletion and RNA missplicing contribute to neuronal vulnerability from loss of TDP-43. Nature Neuroscience. 2011;**14**(4):459-468

[79] Watanabe S et al. ALS-linked TDP-43(M337V) knock-in mice exhibit splicing deregulation without neurodegeneration. Molecular Brain. 2020;**13**(1):8

[80] Wang HY et al. Structural diversity and functional implications of the eukaryotic TDP gene family. Genomics. 2004;**83**(1):130-139

[81] Dreyfuss G et al. hnRNP proteins and the biogenesis of mRNA. Annual Review of Biochemistry. 1993;**62**:289-321

[82] Buratti E et al. TDP-43 binds heterogeneous nuclear ribonucleoprotein a/B through its C-terminal tail: An important region for the inhibition of cystic fibrosis transmembrane conductance regulator exon 9 splicing. The Journal of Biological Chemistry. 2005;**280**(45):37572-37584

[83] Kashima T, Manley JL. A negative element in SMN2 exon 7 inhibits splicing in spinal muscular atrophy. Nature Genetics. 2003;**34**(4):460-463

[84] Buvoli M et al. Alternative splicing in the human gene for the core protein A1 generates another hnRNP protein. The EMBO Journal. 1990;**9**(4):1229-1235

[85] Bekenstein U, Soreq H. Heterogeneous nuclear ribonucleoprotein A1 in health and neurodegenerative disease: From structural insights to post-transcriptional regulatory roles. Molecular and Cellular Neurosciences. 2013;**56**:436-446

[86] Deshaies JE et al. TDP-43 regulates the alternative splicing of hnRNP A1 to yield an aggregation-prone variant in amyotrophic lateral sclerosis. Brain. 2018;**141**(5):1320-1333

[87] Honda H et al. Loss of hnRNPA1 in ALS spinal cord motor neurons with TDP-43-positive inclusions. Neuropathology. 2015;**35**(1):37-43

[88] Jiang LL et al. The N-terminal dimerization is required for TDP-43 splicing activity. Scientific Reports. 2017;7(1):6196

[89] Mompean M et al. Point mutations in the N-terminal domain of transactive response DNA-binding protein 43 kDa (TDP-43) compromise its stability,

dimerization, and functions. The Journal of Biological Chemistry. 2017;**292**(28):11992-12006

[90] Chen HJ et al. RRM adjacent TARDBP mutations disrupt RNA binding and enhance TDP-43 proteinopathy. Brain. 2019;**142**(12):3753-3770

[91] French RL et al. Detection of TAR DNA-binding protein 43 (TDP-43) oligomers as initial intermediate species during aggregate formation. The Journal of Biological Chemistry. 2019;**294**(17):6696-6709

[92] Kawahara Y, Mieda-Sato A. TDP-43 promotes microRNA biogenesis as a component of the Drosha and dicer complexes. Proceedings of the National Academy of Sciences of the United States of America. 2012;**109**(9):3347-3352

[93] Fan Z, Chen X, Chen R. Transcriptome-wide analysis of TDP-43 binding small RNAs identifies miR-NID1 (miR-8485), a novel miRNA that represses NRXN1 expression. Genomics. 2014;**103**(1):76-82

[94] Tollervey JR et al. Characterizing the RNA targets and position-dependent splicing regulation by TDP-43. Nature Neuroscience. 2011;**14**(4):452-458

[95] Beltran M, Garcia de Herreros A. Antisense non-coding RNAs and regulation of gene transcription. Transcription. 2016;7(2):39-43

[96] Liu X et al. Long non-coding RNA gadd7 interacts with TDP-43 and regulates Cdk6 mRNA decay. The EMBO Journal. 2012;**31**(23):4415-4427

[97] Anderson P, Kedersha N. Stress granules: The Tao of RNA triage. Trends in Biochemical Sciences. 2008;**33**(3):141-150

[98] Guil S, Long JC, Caceres JF. hnRNP A1 relocalization to the stress granules reflects a role in the stress response. Molecular and Cellular Biology. 2006;**26**(15):5744-5758

[99] Dewey CM et al. TDP-43 is directed to stress granules by sorbitol, a novel physiological osmotic and oxidative stressor. Molecular and Cellular Biology. 2011;**31**(5):1098-1108

[100] Aulas A, Stabile S, Vande Velde C. Endogenous TDP-43, but not FUS, contributes to stress granule assembly via G3BP. Molecular Neurodegeneration. 2012;7:54

[101] Mackenzie IR et al. TIA1 mutations in amyotrophic lateral sclerosis and Frontotemporal dementia promote phase separation and Alter stress granule dynamics. Neuron. 2017;**95**(4):808-816.e9

[102] Khalfallah Y et al. TDP-43 regulation of stress granule dynamics in neurodegenerative disease-relevant cell types. Scientific Reports. 2018;**8**(1):7551

[103] Aulas A et al. G3BP1 promotes stress-induced RNA granule interactions to preserve polyadenylated mRNA. The Journal of Cell Biology. 2015;**209**(1):73-84

[104] McDonald KK et al. TAR DNA-binding protein 43 (TDP-43) regulates stress granule dynamics via differential regulation of G3BP and TIA-1. Human Molecular Genetics. 2011;**20**(7):1400-1410

[105] Orru S et al. Reduced stress granule formation and cell death in fibroblasts with the A382T mutation of TARDBP gene: Evidence for loss of TDP-43 nuclear function. Human Molecular Genetics. 2016;**25**(20):4473-4483

[106] Gasset-Rosa F et al. Cytoplasmic TDP-43 De-mixing independent of stress granules drives inhibition of nuclear import, loss of nuclear

TDP-43, and cell death. Neuron. 2019;**102**(2):339-357.e7

[107] Hans F, Glasebach H, Kahle PJ. Multiple distinct pathways lead to hyperubiquitylated insoluble TDP-43 protein independent of its translocation into stress granules. The Journal of Biological Chemistry. Jan 17 2020;**295**(3):673-689

[108] Fang MY et al. Small-molecule modulation of TDP-43 recruitment to stress granules prevents persistent TDP-43 accumulation in ALS/FTD. Neuron. 2019;**103**(5):802-819.e11

[109] Chen Y, Cohen TJ. Aggregation of the nucleic acid-binding protein TDP-43 occurs via distinct routes that are coordinated with stress granule formation. The Journal of Biological Chemistry. 2019;**294**(10):3696-3706

[110] Vagnozzi AN, Pratico D. Endosomal sorting and trafficking, the retromer complex and neurodegeneration. Molecular Psychiatry. 2019;**24**(6):857-868

[111] Bouchet J et al. Rab11-FIP3 regulation of Lck Endosomal traffic controls TCR signal transduction. Journal of Immunology. 2017;**198**(7):2967-2978

[112] Touchot N, Chardin P, Tavitian A. Four additional members of the ras gene superfamily isolated by an oligonucleotide strategy: Molecular cloning of YPT-related cDNAs from a rat brain library. Proceedings of the National Academy of Sciences of the United States of America. 1987;**84**(23):8210-8214

[113] Cai H, Reinisch K, Ferro-Novick S. Coats, tethers, Rabs, and SNAREs work together to mediate the intracellular destination of a transport vesicle. Developmental Cell. 2007;**12**(5):671-682

[114] Grosshans BL, Ortiz D, Novick P. Rabs and their effectors: Achieving specificity in membrane traffic. Proceedings of the National Academy of Sciences of the United States of America. 2006;**103**(32):11821-11827

[115] Takahashi S et al. Rab11 regulates exocytosis of recycling vesicles at the plasma membrane. Journal of Cell Science. 2012;**125**(Pt 17):4049-4057

[116] Goldenring JR. Recycling endosomes. Current Opinion in Cell Biology. 2015;**35**:117-122

[117] Bucci C, Alifano P, Cogli L. The role of Rab proteins in neuronal cells and in the trafficking of neurotrophin receptors. Membranes. 2014;**4**(4):642-677

[118] Deshpande M et al. Role of BMP receptor traffic in synaptic growth defects in an ALS model. Molecular Biology of the Cell. 2016;**27**(19):2898-2910

[119] Schwenk BM et al. TDP-43 loss of function inhibits endosomal trafficking and alters trophic signaling in neurons. The EMBO Journal. 2016;**35**(21):2350-2370

[120] Tiwari AK, Roy JK. Mutation in Rab11 results in abnormal organization of ommatidial cells and activation of JNK signaling in the drosophila eye. European Journal of Cell Biology. 2009;**88**(8):445-460

[121] Bhuin T, Roy JK. Rab11 regulates JNK and Raf/MAPK-ERK signalling pathways during drosophila wing development. Cell Biology International. 2010;**34**(11):1113-1118

[122] Li W et al. Heat shock-induced phosphorylation of TAR DNA-binding protein 43 (TDP-43) by MAPK/ERK kinase regulates TDP-43 function.

The Journal of Biological Chemistry. 2017;**292**(12):5089-5100

[123] Mitra J, Hegde PM, Hegde ML. Loss of endosomal recycling factor RAB11 coupled with complex regulation of MAPK/ERK/AKT signaling in postmortem spinal cord specimens of sporadic amyotrophic lateral sclerosis patients. Molecular Brain. 2019;**12**(1):55

[124] Winter JN, Jefferson LS, Kimball SR. ERK and Akt signaling pathways function through parallel mechanisms to promote mTORC1 signaling. American Journal of Physiology. Cell Physiology. 2011;**300**(5):C1172-C1180

[125] Breda C et al. Rab11 modulates alpha-synuclein-mediated defects in synaptic transmission and behaviour. Human Molecular Genetics. 2015;**24**(4):1077-1091

[126] Steinert JR et al. Rab11 rescues synaptic dysfunction and behavioural deficits in a drosophila model of Huntington's disease. Human Molecular Genetics. 2012;**21**(13):2912-2922

[127] Li X et al. Disruption of Rab11 activity in a knock-in mouse model of Huntington's disease. Neurobiology of Disease. 2009;**36**(2):374-383

[128] Farg MA et al. C9ORF72, implicated in amytrophic lateral sclerosis and frontotemporal dementia, regulates endosomal trafficking. Human Molecular Genetics. 2017;**26**(20):4093-4094

[129] Cheung K et al. Rho guanine nucleotide exchange factor (RGNEF) is a prosurvival factor under stress conditions. Molecular and Cellular Neurosciences. 2017;**82**:88-95

[130] Droppelmann CA et al. Rho guanine nucleotide exchange factor is an NFL mRNA destabilizing factor that forms cytoplasmic inclusions in amyotrophic lateral sclerosis. Neurobiology of Aging. 2013;**34**(1):248-262

[131] Keller BA et al. Co-aggregation of RNA binding proteins in ALS spinal motor neurons: Evidence of a common pathogenic mechanism. Acta Neuropathologica. 2012;**124**(5):733-747

[132] Utani K et al. Emergence of micronuclei and their effects on the fate of cells under replication stress. PLoS One. 2010;**5**(4):e10089

[133] Kiraly G et al. Micronucleus formation during chromatin condensation and under apoptotic conditions. Apoptosis. 2017;**22**(2):207-219

[134] Xu B et al. Replication stress induces micronuclei comprising of aggregated DNA double-strand breaks. PLoS One. 2011;**6**(4):e18618

[135] Droppelmann CA et al. TDP-43 aggregation inside micronuclei reveals a potential mechanism for protein inclusion formation in ALS. Scientific Reports. 2019;**9**(1):19928

[136] Ou SH et al. Cloning and characterization of a novel cellular protein, TDP-43, that binds to human immunodeficiency virus type 1 TAR DNA sequence motifs. Journal of Virology. 1995;**69**(6):3584-3596

[137] Nehls J et al. HIV-1 replication in human immune cells is independent of TAR DNA binding protein 43 (TDP-43) expression. PLoS One. 2014;**9**(8):e105478

[138] Furukawa Y et al. A molecular mechanism realizing sequence-specific recognition of nucleic acids by TDP-43. Scientific Reports. 2016;**6**:20576

[139] Ayala YM, Misteli T, Baralle FE. TDP-43 regulates retinoblastoma protein phosphorylation through the repression of cyclin-dependent

kinase 6 expression. Proceedings of the National Academy of Sciences of the United States of America. 2008;**105**(10):3785-3789

[140] Lalmansingh AS, Urekar CJ, Reddi PP. TDP-43 is a transcriptional repressor: The testis-specific mouse acrv1 gene is a TDP-43 target in vivo. The Journal of Biological Chemistry. 2011;**286**(13):10970-10982

[141] Abhyankar MM, Urekar C, Reddi PP. A novel CpG-free vertebrate insulator silences the testis-specific SP-10 gene in somatic tissues: Role for TDP-43 in insulator function. The Journal of Biological Chemistry. 2007;**282**(50):36143-36154

[142] Acharya KK et al. Cis-requirement for the maintenance of round spermatid-specific transcription. Developmental Biology. 2006;**295**(2):781-790

[143] Kitamura A et al. Analysis of the substrate recognition state of TDP-43 to single-stranded DNA using fluorescence correlation spectroscopy. Biochemistry and Biophysics Reports. 2018;**14**:58-63

[144] Kuo PH et al. The crystal structure of TDP-43 RRM1-DNA complex reveals the specific recognition for UG- and TG-rich nucleic acids. Nucleic Acids Research. 2014;**42**(7):4712-4722

[145] Qin H et al. TDP-43 N terminus encodes a novel ubiquitin-like fold and its unfolded form in equilibrium that can be shifted by binding to ssDNA. Proceedings of the National Academy of Sciences of the United States of America. 2014;**111**(52):18619-18624

[146] Mitra J et al. Motor neuron disease-associated loss of nuclear TDP-43 is linked to DNA double-strand break repair defects. Proceedings of the National Academy of Sciences of the United States of America. 2019;**116**(10):4696-4705

[147] Vasquez V et al. Chromatin-bound oxidized alpha-Synuclein causes Strand breaks in neuronal genomes in in vitro models of Parkinson's disease. Journal of Alzheimer's Disease. 2017;**60**(s1):S133-s150

[148] Hou Y et al. NAD(+) supplementation normalizes key Alzheimer's features and DNA damage responses in a new AD mouse model with introduced DNA repair deficiency. Proceedings of the National Academy of Sciences of the United States of America. 2018;**115**(8):E1876-e1885

[149] Madabhushi R et al. Activity-induced DNA breaks govern the expression of neuronal early-response genes. Cell. 2015;**161**(7):1592-1605

[150] Su Y, Ming GL, Song H. DNA damage and repair regulate neuronal gene expression. Cell Research. 2015;**25**(9):993-994

[151] Freibaum BD et al. Global analysis of TDP-43 interacting proteins reveals strong association with RNA splicing and translation machinery. Journal of Proteome Research. 2010;**9**(2):1104-1120

[152] Nagase M et al. Increased oxidative stress in patients with amyotrophic lateral sclerosis and the effect of edaravone administration. Redox Report. 2016;**21**(3):104-112

[153] Niedzielska E et al. Oxidative stress in neurodegenerative diseases. Molecular Neurobiology. 2016;**53**(6):4094-4125

[154] Kabuta C et al. 4-Hydroxynonenal induces persistent insolubilization of TDP-43 and alters its intracellular localization. Biochemical and Biophysical Research Communications. 2015;**463**(1-2):82-87

[155] Zinszner H, Albalat R, Ron D. A novel effector domain from the

RNA-binding protein TLS or EWS is required for oncogenic transformation by CHOP. Genes & Development. 1994;**8**(21):2513-2526

[156] Caragounis A et al. Zinc induces depletion and aggregation of endogenous TDP-43. Free Radical Biology & Medicine. 2010;**48**(9):1152-1161

[157] Hegde ML et al. Scaffold attachment factor a (SAF-A) and Ku temporally regulate repair of radiation-induced clustered genome lesions. Oncotarget. 2016;**7**(34):54430-54444

[158] Hegde ML et al. Enhancement of NEIL1 protein-initiated oxidized DNA base excision repair by heterogeneous nuclear ribonucleoprotein U (hnRNP-U) via direct interaction. The Journal of Biological Chemistry. 2012;**287**(41):34202-34211

Chapter 2

Molecular Basis of DNA Repair Defects in FUS-Associated ALS: Implications of a New Paradigm and Its Potential as Therapeutic Target

Haibo Wang and Muralidhar L. Hegde

Abstract

Amyotrophic lateral sclerosis (ALS) is a progressive motor neuron disorder, characterized by a diverse etiopathology. While ALS is predominantly sporadic, mutations in one or more of a dozen risk factors have been linked to approximately 10% of familial ALS patients. The multifunctional RNA/DNA-binding protein fused in sarcoma (FUS) is one such protein whose autosomal dominant missense mutations were identified in a subset of familial and sporadic ALS patients. Initial studies linked FUS with both RNA-related and genome maintenance functions, yet the mechanisms and potential implications to neurodegeneration were not completely understood. We recently identified a novel function of FUS in repairing single-strand break (SSB) in the genome. FUS directly interacts and recruits XRCC1/DNA Ligase IIIα (LigIII) to DNA oxidative damage sites in a PARP1 activity-dependent manner, which facilitates optimal oxidative genome damage repair. Besides, FUS regulates DNA strand break sealing by enhancing ligation activity of LigIII. The mutation of FUS induces accumulation of oxidative DNA damage as well as DNA repair deficiency in ALS patients. The novel findings provide insights into a previously undescribed mechanism of DNA repair defect in FUS-associated neurodegeneration, and raise the pentientials of developing neuroprotective therapies by targeting DNA break ligating defects.

Keywords: FUS, neurodegeneration, DNA repair, oxidative genome damage, XRCC1-DNA ligase III

1. Fused in sarcoma (FUS): pathophysiology and links to familial and sporadic ALS

1.1 FUS and its physiological functions

The FUS/TLS (Fused in sarcoma Protein/Translocated in liposarcoma) gene encodes a 526-amino acid protein that belongs to the TET (TAF15, EWS, and TLS) family, which is implicated in multiple aspects of RNA metabolism. The FUS gene was initially identified as an oncogene in multiple cancers. FUS fuses with the transcription repressor C/EBP homologous protein 10 (CHOP) in myxoid liposarcomas. It was identified for its role as an activator of ETS-related gene (ERG) in acute myeloid leukemia [1, 2] and in Ewing's sarcoma tumors [3]. Subsequently, mutations in FUS were linked to motor neuron diseases, amyotrophic lateral sclerosis (ALS), and frontotemporal dementia (FTD) [4, 5].

FUS protein is ubiquitously expressed in both the nucleus and cytoplasm of many cell types; however, it is predominantly found in the nucleus of glial cells and neurons in the central nervous system. A small fraction of FUS shuttles between the nucleus and cytoplasm under various stimuli, for example, sodium arsenite-induced oxidative stress [6, 7]. A previous study revealed that FUS binds RNA *in vivo* to engage in nucleo-cytoplasmic shuttling [8]. Another study showed that FUS is localized to dendritic spines as an RNA-protein complex and associates with mRNA encoding an actin-stabilizer protein, which indicates a regulatory role of FUS in actin/cytoskeleton processes in dendrites [9]. Interestingly, in response to stress-induced by sorbitol, FUS redistributes to the cytoplasm and localizes to cytoplasmic stress granules [10], a complex comprised of mRNA, ribosomes, RNA-binding proteins, transcription factors and nucleases that form in response to induced stress, such as oxidative stress and heat shock to maintain the stability of selected mRNAs and protein activities [11, 12]. The redistribution of FUS on stress granules is regulated by posttranslational modification, methylation, and highly related with cell survival from the stress [10]. FUS protein contains an SYGQ-rich region at its N terminal, followed by a RGG box (RGG1), an RRM motif, a second RGG box (RGG2), a zinc finger (ZnF) motif, and a third RGG box (RGG3). The C-terminus contains a nonclassical nuclear localization signal (NLS) with conserved proline and tyrosine residues (PY-NLS). The 13 terminal amino acids (514–526) containing the NLS sequence were shown to be necessary, but not sufficient, for nuclear import of FUS [13]. FUS can bind with RNA and both single-stranded (ss) as well as double-stranded (ds) DNA [14]. FUS is associated with multiple roles in RNA processing, including splicing, transcription, and transport. Studies have highlighted that FUS has a transcriptional regulatory role in global or specialized components of transcriptional machinery [15]. A Clip-seq based study revealed that FUS regulates alternative splicing of pre-mRNAs and processing of long-intron containing transcripts, and the RNAs targeted by FUS are associated with neurogenesis and gene expression regulation; interestingly, some of FUS' mRNA targets are involved in DNA damage response and repair pathways [16].

1.2 FUS is mutated in both familial and sporadic ALS

The prevalence of ALS has been observed to be non-uniform geographically but ranges between 0.6 and 3.8 per 100,000 population worldwide. The rate of ALS incidence appears to be rising according to the recent epidemiological studies, despite the geographical differences [17]. Notably, the incidence and prevalence of ALS are greater in men than in women [18]. It has been reported that the male: female ratio is between 1 and 3 and changes in an age-dependent manner [19]. In approximately 90% of ALS cases the cause is unknown, and, as such, they are considered sporadic (SALS); while, around 10% of ALS patients have a clear family history (FALS). In 2009, two independent studies identified that FUS R521 is mutated in FALS cases and that mutation is characterized pathologically with enhanced cytoplasmic inclusions of FUS and motor neuron degeneration [4, 5]. FUS mutations have also been linked to cases of SALS [20–22]. The FUS gene is composed of 15 exons and most mutations are clustered in exon15. Exon15 encodes the NLS domain, implying a possible involvement of its nuclear import defects. These mutations/truncations include 495X, R521C/G/H/L/S, R522G, P525L, and so on. R521 is the most commonly mutated site in ALS, whereas P525 mutations are highly related with early onset and severe progress of ALS [23–25]. Mutations also occur in domains other than NLS. For example, G187S within Gly-rich domain, G399V in RGG domain, and P431L in ZnF domain [26], which is believed to induce functional defects of FUS. Autosomal dominant mutations in the gene encoding the FUS protein have been detected in approximately 5% of FALS patients and a small subset (~1%) of SALS cases.

1.3 FUS pathology in FTD

It is important to note that many ALS patients (36–51%) also exhibit cognitive impairment, with about 20% developing FTD, also called frontotemporal lobar degeneration (FTLD) [27], a disorder characterized by cognitive, behavioral, and linguistic dysfunction. The reverse is also seen, wherein patients with FTD can develop ALS [28]. FTD accounts for 10–15% of dementias, making it the second most common type of dementia for people under the age of 65, after Alzheimer's disease. The overlap between ALS and FTD indicates a likely common molecular basis between FUS and cognitive deficits. After the discovery of FUS mutation in ALS, a novel subtype of FTD with FUS pathology was identified, although no FUS mutation was seen [29]. In 2010, Oriane Broustal et al. identified three exonic FUS variants, c. 1562G > A (p.Arg521His), c. 1566G > A (p.Arg522Arg), and c.188A > G (pAsn63Ser) from 317 patients including 144 patients with familial FTD and 173 patients with FTD-ALS. Interestingly, the three variants were found only in patients with both FTD and ALS [27].

2. Multifaceted role of FUS in RNA and DNA transactions

The molecular mechanisms of FUS-ALS are complex and ambiguous, typically described by both loss of function and gain of toxicity hypotheses. Although controversial, loss of function is not entirely supported by animal models: FUS knockout mice and zebrafish do not develop ALS-like phenotypes [30–32]. As mentioned in the previous section, FUS plays multiple roles in RNA metabolism. In fact, thousands of RNA targets have been identified that bind to FUS in various cell lines and brain tissue from both patients and animal models [33]. The dysregulation and disturbance of RNA processing are considered to be one mechanism that leads to neurodegeneration. Depletion of FUS in mouse nervous system has been shown to alter the levels of splicing of over 950 mRNAs [34]; FUS knockout in neuroblastoma cells disturbs the splicing of more than 400 introns [35]. Expression of FUS P525L mutant was shown to inhibit splicing of minor introns by trapping U11 and U12 small nuclear RNAs (snRNAs) in these aggregates [35], and expression of R521G and R522G mutations influence RNA transcription and splicing but in a different way [36]. Besides, mRNA transport and stabilization are also affected by ALS-linked FUS mutations [37, 38].

The majority of the mutations occur in the NLS region of FUS, which induces its cytoplasmic accumulation. The widespread FUS mislocalization has been considered a hallmark of ALS [39]. Mutant, but not the wild-type FUS was shown to be assembled into stress granules in cytoplasm in response to oxidative stress or heat shock [7, 40], which potentially contributes to neurotoxicity by impairing mRNA translation [41, 42]. In fact, mutations in RNA-binding proteins (RBPs) are highly related to ALS. The interaction between mistranslocated FUS and other RBPs was recently investigated. These studies show that the cytoplasmic mislocalization caused by FUS P525L mutation impairs its interaction with other ALS-associated

RBPs including shnRNPA1, hnRNPA2B1, EWSR1, and TAF15, which facilitates the nucleation of toxic cytoplasmic FUS aggregates. In addition, high cytoplasmic FUS levels exhibit defects in protein degradation and reduced protein levels of RBPs, shedding lights on the FUS-ALS pathology linked to the homeostasis of multiple ALS-associated RBPs [43].

2.1 FUS toxicity and impaired DNA damage response (DDR) signaling

In addition to RNA dysregulation, there has been a lot of focus on the genome instability caused by FUS mutation in ALS patients since FUS was first linked to DNA damage repair by multiple studies. In human cells, one major source of genome damage is the reactive oxygen species (ROS) accumulation-induced oxidative stress. ROS that defined as a group of reactive molecules derived from oxygen including but not limited to free radicals (superoxide, O_2^-), hydroxyl radical (·OH), or non-radicals (hydrogen peroxide) can be balanced by various antioxidant systems, while the imbalance between ROS production and antioxidant defenses causes oxidative stress, leading to oxidation of lipid, protein, and DNA in cells [44]. Accumulation of oxidative DNA damge has been linked to multiple neurodegenerative diseases like Parkinson's disease (PD) and Huntington's disease (HD) [45, 46]. In addition to DNA damage, mutation in the genes of specific DNA repair pathways that lead to DNA damage repair (DDR) is another challenge for the central nervous system [47]. For example, nucleotide excision repair (NER) is defective in xeroderma pigmentosum (XP) and Cockayne syndrome (CS), base excision/single-strand break repair (BER/SSBR) defects in ataxia with oculomotor apraxia type 1 (AOA1) [48], spinocerebellar ataxia with axonal neuropathy (SCAN1) [49] and ALS [50], and defective DDR signaling and DNA double-strand break repair (DSBR) in ataxia telangiectasia (A-T) and Nijmegen break-age syndrome. FUS is found to be phosphorylated by DDR proteins ataxia-telangiectasia mutated (ATM) and DNA-dependent protein kinase (DNA-PK) in response to DSB-inducing agents. FUS was identified to interact with histone deacetylase 1 (HDAC1) in primary mouse cortical neurons, and the interaction is believed to modulate the homologous recombination (HR) and non-homologous end joining (NHEJ), two major pathways for DSB repair. Besides, FUS was shown to be recruited at DNA damage tracks induced by microirradiation (MIR) at wavelengths of 405 or 351 nm, in a PARP1-depedent manner and accompanied with PARylation by PARP1 [51–53]. Notably, MIR causes clusters of different types of DNA damage including oxidized base lesions, single-strand breaks (SSBs), and DSBs. It is generally believed that UVA (wavelength between 320 and 400 nm) predominantly induces SSBs via elevated ROS, while UVA may also induce secondary DSBs due to clustered SSBs [54]. Thus, recruitment of FUS at MIR with wavelength of 351 nm suggests its potential role in the repair of SSBs.

2.2 FUS and repair of oxidative genome damage: mechanistic insights

A comprehensive investigation by our group described the mechanistic role of FUS in BER/SSBR, a major pathway to repair oxidative DNA damage. Our study utilized multiple *in vitro* and *in vivo* model systems, including, CRISPR/Cas9-mediated FUS knockout (KO) human embryonic kidney (HEK)293 cells, FALS patient-derived induced pluripotent stem cells (iPSCs) with FUS mutations R521H and P525L, motor neurons induced from these iPSC lines, and ALS patients spinal cord tissues with FUS pathology. We discovered that the DNA integrity is substantially affected in the spinal cord tissues and the motor neurons derived from ALS patients. Both downregulation and pathological mutation of FUS were associated with DNA SSB accumulation and SSBR defects. Finally, we identified that FUS directly interacts with PARP1, XRCC1, and LigIII in response to oxidative stress and FUS facilitates the recruitment of XRCC1/LigIII to DNA damage sites in a PARP1 activity-dependent manner. FUS enhances the ligation activity of LigIII, which is critical for an optimal SSBR in neurons (**Figure 1**). The SSBR deficiency due to ALS-linked FUS mutations can be rescued by the correction of those mutations via Crisper/Cas9 technology [50]. Furthermore, FUS regulates PARP1's PARylation activity in motor neurons and thus could affect neuronal energy metabolism by uncoupling NAD^+/NADH levels.

2.3 FUS-PARP-1 interactions: a new paradigm with diverse implications

During DDR, PARP1 plays an important role in regulating DNA damage repair. In response to DNA damage, PARP1 is self-activated by its auto-PARylation and transfers ADP-ribose to create long and branched poly(ADP-ribose) on target DNA repair proteins to facilitate their recruitment; for example, PARP1 recruits XRCC1 by its PARylation. A study showed that PARP1 likely plays a major role for the poly(ADP-ribose) synthesis induced by alkylating agents, since the amount of poly(ADP-ribose) can be reduced for around 10 folds (from 60 pmol per mg of DNA to 5.85 pmol per mg of DNA) in PARP1 KO cells in the presence of MNNG [55], which activates DNA mismatch repair. Consistantly, PARP1 knockout mice are

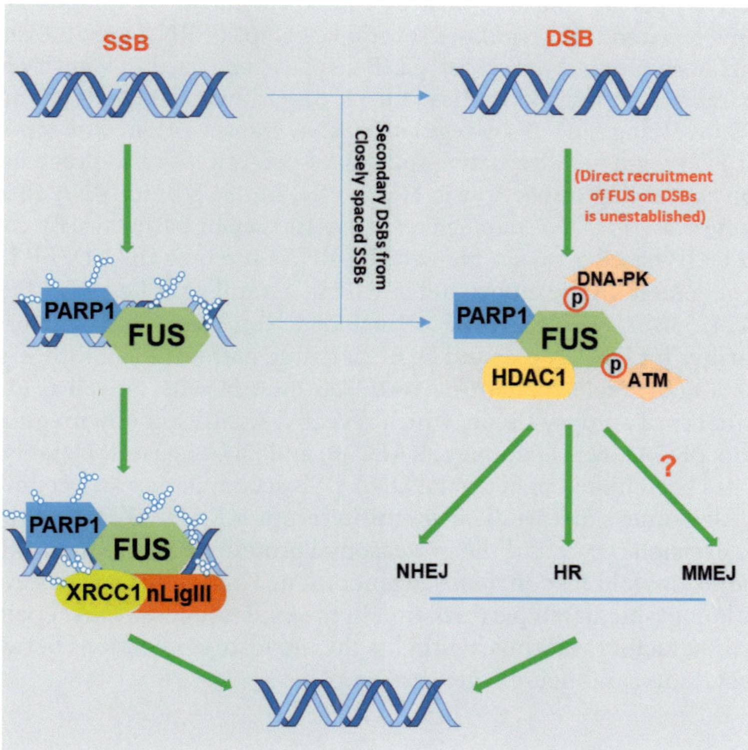

Figure 1.
Model of FUS involving DNA damage response in the nucleus. In response to DNA SSBs, FUS is PARylated and recruited to DNA damage sites by PARP1 and the recruitment facilitates the loading of XRCC1 and nuclear LigIII (nLigIII) complex, where FUS enhances the ligation activity of LigIII for an optimal SSB ligating. While in response to DSB, FUS is associated with HDAC1, which is required for an efficient NHEJ and HR-mediated DSB repair. FUS is also phosphorylated by ATM and DNA-PK, although the underlying mechanism is not known. Due to its role in the functional activation of LigII, which is involved in MMEJ-mediated DSB repair, it is likely that FUS also affects MMEJ, which needs to be investigated.

highly susceptible to DNA damaging agents and are accumulated with DNA strand breaks accompanied with genomic instability in them [56, 57].

In response to DNA damage, FUS is recruited to DNA damage site in a PARP1 activity-dependent manner [51, 52]. FUS directly binds to PAR synthesized by activated PARP1 leading to the formation of damaged DNA-rich compartments contributed by its N-terminal low-complexity domain (LCD) and C-terminal RGG domains, and the compartments are dissociated by the hydrolysis of PAR by PARG [58], which indicates that PAR polymers play an essential role for the recruitment, likely through enhancing the FUS droplet formation [59]. While the activation of PARP1 can induce shuttling of FUS from nucleus to cytoplasm, which in turn enhances FUS aggregate formation and neurodegeneration [58, 60]. Furthermore, like FUS, the other two members in TET family, TAF15 and EWSR1 are also recruited to MIR-induced DNA damage tracks depending on PARP1 activity [53], while the molecular mechanism of the cross-talk between TET family proteins and PARP-1 has not been investigated.

3. Indirect role of FUS in DDR: FUS-directed RNA transactions in DNA repair

Although, recent reports from our group and others demonstrate a complex, but the direct role of FUS in maintaining genome integrity, whether FUS RNA-binding activity plays a role in regulating the expression of DDR factors has not been investigated. FUS regulates several key steps of RNA metabolism that impairs various biological processes. CLIP-seq has been used to identify RNAs that FUS targeted in multiple studies [16, 34, 61–65], which reveals an indirect role of FUS involving in DDR by regulating RNA transcription. One report shows that FUS regulates alternative splicing of pre-mRNAs and processing of long-intron containing transcripts in HeLa cells, and FUS binds RNA encoding proteins important for DNA damage response and repair pathways. By comparing with other CLIP-based assays, a map of FUS RNA targets to DNA DSBR by NHEJ and HR is generated in the report and in which, a number of key DDR factors such as ATM, 53BP1, MRN11, NBS1 are included [16]. We recently performed RT^2 PCR arrays for DNA repair and DDR signaling pathways in CRISPR/cas9 FUS knockout (KO) cells, patient-derived FUS-mutant cells, as well as FUS-ALS patient spinal cord autopsy tissue, which revealed significant downregulation of DDR factors BRCA1, MSH complex, RAD23B, and DNA ligase 4. Notably, BRCA1 depletion has been linked to neuronal DNA DSB accumulation and cognitive defects in Alzheimer's disease. The ubiquitin receptor RAD23 functions both in nucleotide excision repair and the proteasomal protein clearance pathway and is thus linked to amyloid load in neurodegeneration. This study provides evidence of FUS pathology-mediated perturbation in the expression of DNA repair and DDR signaling factors and thus highlights the intricate connections between FUS, genome instability, and neurodegeneration.

4. Conclusions and perspectives

As early as 1982, the defective DNA repair and its possible role in ALS pathology was first proposed by Bradley et al. [66], where they hypothesize that abnormal DNA in ALS may arise from a deficiency of an isozyme of a DNA repair factor. Subsequently, growing evidence suggests that defective DNA repair is a common feature of not only ALS but also several other neurodegenerative diseases, underscoring the needs of studying the implications of unrepaired DNA damage in neurons affected by neurodegeneration [67], which may lead to novel therapeutic strategies.

Our recent studies made a critical breakthrough in this direction by first time shedding lights on the molecular insights into the involvement of ALS and FTD-associated FUS and other RNA/DNA-binding proteins in specific DNA repair failure mechanisms, such as DNA ligation deficiency. While this study suggests a potential for DNA ligase complementation strategy, several key questions should be addressed to develop DNA repair-based interventions for ALS. These are: (1) The role of FUS in mitochondrial genome stability maintaining. The linkage between FUS and mitochondrial integrity has been established by a number of studies. Deng et al. demonstrated interactions between FUS and two mitochondrial proteins, mitochondrial chaperonin HSP60 and ATP synthase beta subunit ATP5B, in different studies. HSP60 mediates the translocation of FUS into mitochondria, and downregulating of HSP60 rescues mitochondrial defects and neurodegenerative phenotypes in FUS transgenic flies. While interaction between FUS and ATP5B indicates a involvement of FUS in the dysregulation of mitochondrial ATP synthesis: expression of wild-type or FUS P525L mutant disrupts the formation of the mitochondrial ATP synthase supercomplexes and suppresses the activity of ATP synthase, resulting in mitochondrial cristae loss followed by mitochondrial fragmentation [68, 69]. Nakaya and Maragkakis et al. found that expression of human FUS R495X in mouse embryonic stem cell-differentiated neurons disturbs the translation efficiency of mitochondria-associated genes and results in significant reduction of mitochondrial size [70]. Although ALS-FUS has been linked with the dysfunction of mitochondria, the role of FUS in mitochondrial genome integrity has not been explored. (2) The role of FUS in microhomology-mediated end joining (MMEJ) repair. We have established a relationship between FUS and XRCC1/LigIII, which is required for an optimal SSBR. While LigIII, together with XRCC1 and PARP1, also participates in the MMEJ-mediated DSB repair pathway, the role of which in primary neurons is unknown (**Figure 1**). We hypothesized that the MMEJ contributes DSBR in motor neurons and the loss of FUS may affect MMEJ and lead to genomic instability, which we are currently pursuing. (3) The role of FUS in maintaining genome integrity in astrocytes. Recent studies have shown that expression of ALS-linked mutant FUS and other ALS causative factors in astrocytes induces motor neuron death [71–73]. It will, therefore, be critical to investigate FUS toxicity-induced ligation activity defects in astrocytes and the collateral influence on motor neurons. (4) Whether DNA ligase I (LigI) rescues FUS mutant-mediated LigIII defects. Mammalian cells express three DNA ligases including ligase IV (LigIV), LigIII, and LigI. LigIV specifically participates in NHEJ-mediated DSB repair; LigIII has nuclear and mitochondrial isoforms. Both the nuclear and mitochondrial isoforms have ~98% similarity and function in BER/single-strand break repair (SSBR); LigI has been shown to functionally overlap with LigIII and is believed a back-up of LigIII, however, the level of LigI expression in non-cycling, postmitotic cells like neurons is negligible due to lack of replication-associated repair. Very likely, the induction of LigI into motor neurons with FUS pathology can rescue the LigIII ligation activity defects caused by FUS mutation.

Addressing these critical follow-up questions is an unmet need in the FUS-ALS field, which will help to develop a mechanism-based DNA-repair-targeted therapy. With recent emerging studies, the stage is set for such a paradigm shift.

Acknowledgements

The research was supported by grants from the National Institute of Neurological Disorders and Stroke (NINDS) of the National Institute of Health (NIH) under the award numbers R01NS088645, RF1NS112719 and the Houston Methodist Research Institute funds. The content is solely the responsibility of the authors and does not necessarily represent the official views of the funding agencies.

Author details

Haibo Wang[1,2*] and Muralidhar L. Hegde[1,2,3*]

1 Department of Radiation Oncology, Houston Methodist Research Institute, Houston, TX, USA

2 Department of Neurosurgery, Center for Neuroregeneration, Houston Methodist Neurological Institute, Institute of Academic Medicine, Houston Methodist Hospital, Houston, TX, USA

3 Weill Medical College, New York, NY, USA

*Address all correspondence to: hwang@houstonmethodist.org and mlhegde@houstonmethodist.org

References

[1] Ichikawa H, Shimizu K, Hayashi Y, Ohki M. An RNA-binding protein gene, TLS/FUS, is fused to ERG in human myeloid leukemia with t(16,21) chromosomal translocation. Cancer Research. 1994;**54**(11):2865-2868

[2] Panagopoulos I, Aman P, Fioretos T, Hoglund M, Johansson B, Mandahl N, et al. Fusion of the FUS gene with ERG in acute myeloid leukemia with t(16,21) (p11;q22). Genes, Chromosomes & Cancer. 1994;**11**(4):256-262

[3] Shing DC, McMullan DJ, Roberts P, Smith K, Chin SF, Nicholson J, et al. FUS/ERG gene fusions in Ewing's tumors. Cancer Research. 2003;**63**(15):4568-4576

[4] Kwiatkowski TJ Jr, Bosco DA, Leclerc AL, Tamrazian E, Vanderburg CR, Russ C, et al. Mutations in the FUS/TLS gene on chromosome 16 cause familial amyotrophic lateral sclerosis. Science. 2009;**323**(5918):1205-1208

[5] Vance C, Rogelj B, Hortobagyi T, De Vos KJ, Nishimura AL, Sreedharan J, et al. Mutations in FUS, an RNA processing protein, cause familial amyotrophic lateral sclerosis type 6. Science. 2009;**323**(5918):1208-1211

[6] Vance C, Scotter EL, Nishimura AL, Troakes C, Mitchell JC, Kathe C, et al. ALS mutant FUS disrupts nuclear localization and sequesters wild-type FUS within cytoplasmic stress granules. Human Molecular Genetics. 2013;**22**(13):2676-2688

[7] Gal J, Zhang J, Kwinter DM, Zhai J, Jia H, Jia J, et al. Nuclear localization sequence of FUS and induction of stress granules by ALS mutants. Neurobiology of Aging. 2011;**32**(12):e2327-e2340

[8] Zinszner H, Sok J, Immanuel D, Yin Y, Ron D. TLS (FUS) binds RNA in vivo and engages in nucleo-cytoplasmic shuttling. Journal of Cell Science. 1997;**110**(Pt 15):1741-1750

[9] Fujii R, Takumi T. TLS facilitates transport of mRNA encoding an actin-stabilizing protein to dendritic spines. Journal of Cell Science. 2005;**118**(Pt 24): 5755-5765

[10] Sama RR, Ward CL, Kaushansky LJ, Lemay N, Ishigaki S, Urano F, et al. FUS/TLS assembles into stress granules and is a prosurvival factor during hyperosmolar stress. Journal of Cellular Physiology. 2013;**228**(11):2222-2231

[11] Anderson P, Kedersha N. Stress granules. Current Biology. 2009;**19**(10):R397-R398

[12] Kedersha N, Anderson P. Stress granules: Sites of mRNA triage that regulate mRNA stability and translatability. Biochemical Society Transactions. 2002;**30**(Pt 6):963-969

[13] Dormann D, Rodde R, Edbauer D, Bentmann E, Fischer I, Hruscha A, et al. ALS-associated fused in sarcoma (FUS) mutations disrupt transportin-mediated nuclear import. The EMBO Journal. 2010;**29**(16):2841-2857

[14] Tan AY, Manley JL. The TET family of proteins: Functions and roles in disease. Journal of Molecular Cell Biology. 2009;**1**(2):82-92

[15] Masuda A, Takeda J, Ohno K. FUS-mediated regulation of alternative RNA processing in neurons: Insights from global transcriptome analysis. Wiley Interdisciplinary Reviews: RNA. 2016;**7**(3):330-340

[16] Zhou Y, Liu S, Ozturk A, Hicks GG. FUS-regulated RNA metabolism and DNA damage repair: Implications for amyotrophic lateral sclerosis and frontotemporal dementia pathogenesis. Rare Disease. 2014;**2**:e29515

[17] Longinetti E, Fang F. Epidemiology of amyotrophic lateral sclerosis: An update of recent literature. Current Opinion in Neurology. 2019;**32**(5):771-776

[18] McCombe PA, Henderson RD. Effects of gender in amyotrophic lateral sclerosis. Gender Medicine. 2010;7(6):557-570

[19] Manjaly ZR, Scott KM, Abhinav K, Wijesekera L, Ganesalingam J, Goldstein LH, et al. The sex ratio in amyotrophic lateral sclerosis: A population based study. Amyotrophic Lateral Sclerosis. 2010;**11**(5):439-442

[20] Lai SL, Abramzon Y, Schymick JC, Stephan DA, Dunckley T, Dillman A, et al. FUS mutations in sporadic amyotrophic lateral sclerosis. Neurobiology of Aging. 2011;**32**(3):e551-e554

[21] Rademakers R, Stewart H, Dejesus-Hernandez M, Krieger C, Graff-Radford N, Fabros M, et al. Fus gene mutations in familial and sporadic amyotrophic lateral sclerosis. Muscle & Nerve. 2010;**42**(2):170-176

[22] Zou ZY, Peng Y, Feng XH, Wang XN, Sun Q, Liu MS, et al. Screening of the FUS gene in familial and sporadic amyotrophic lateral sclerosis patients of Chinese origin. European Journal of Neurology. 2012;**19**(7):977-983

[23] Conte A, Lattante S, Zollino M, Marangi G, Luigetti M, Del Grande A, et al. P525L FUS mutation is consistently associated with a severe form of juvenile amyotrophic lateral sclerosis. Neuromuscular Disorders. 2012;**22**(1):73-75

[24] Eura N, Sugie K, Suzuki N, Kiriyama T, Izumi T, Shimakura N, et al. A juvenile sporadic amyotrophic lateral sclerosis case with P525L mutation in the FUS gene: A rare co-occurrence of autism spectrum disorder and tremor. Journal of the Neurological Sciences. 2019;**398**:67-68

[25] Baumer D, Hilton D, Paine SM, Turner MR, Lowe J, Talbot K, et al. Juvenile ALS with basophilic inclusions is a FUS proteinopathy with FUS mutations. Neurology. 2010;**75**(7):611-618

[26] Harrison AF, Shorter J. RNA-binding proteins with prion-like domains in health and disease. The Biochemical Journal. 2017;**474**(8):1417-1438

[27] Broustal O, Camuzat A, Guillot-Noel L, Guy N, Millecamps S, Deffond D, et al. FUS mutations in frontotemporal lobar degeneration with amyotrophic lateral sclerosis. Journal of Alzheimer's Disease. 2010;**22**(3):765-769

[28] Lipton AM, White CL 3rd, Bigio EH. Frontotemporal lobar degeneration with motor neuron disease-type inclusions predominates in 76 cases of frontotemporal degeneration. Acta Neuropathologica. 2004;**108**(5):379-385

[29] Neumann M, Rademakers R, Roeber S, Baker M, Kretzschmar HA, Mackenzie IR. A new subtype of frontotemporal lobar degeneration with FUS pathology. Brain. 2009;**132** (Pt 11):2922-2931

[30] Kino Y, Washizu C, Kurosawa M, Yamada M, Miyazaki H, Akagi T, et al. FUS/TLS deficiency causes behavioral and pathological abnormalities distinct from amyotrophic lateral sclerosis. Acta Neuropathologica Communications. 2015;**3**:24

[31] Lebedeva S, de Jesus Domingues AM, Butter F, Ketting RF. Characterization of genetic loss-of-function of FUS in zebrafish. RNA Biology. 2017;**14**(1):29-35

[32] Sharma A, Lyashchenko AK, Lu L, Nasrabady SE, Elmaleh M, Mendelsohn M, et al. ALS-associated mutant FUS induces selective motor neuron degeneration through toxic gain of function. Nature Communications. 2016;7:10465

[33] Butti Z, Patten SA. RNA dysregulation in amyotrophic lateral sclerosis. Frontiers in Genetics. 2018;**9**:712

[34] Lagier-Tourenne C, Polymenidou M, Hutt KR, Vu AQ, Baughn M, Huelga SC, et al. Divergent roles of ALS-linked proteins FUS/TLS and TDP-43 intersect in processing long pre-mRNAs. Nature Neuroscience. 2012;**15**(11):1488-1497

[35] Reber S, Stettler J, Filosa G, Colombo M, Jutzi D, Lenzken SC, et al. Minor intron splicing is regulated by FUS and affected by ALS-associated FUS mutants. The EMBO Journal. 2016;**35**(14):1504-1521

[36] van Blitterswijk M, Wang ET, Friedman BA, Keagle PJ, Lowe P, Leclerc AL, et al. Characterization of FUS mutations in amyotrophic lateral sclerosis using RNA-Seq. PLoS One. 2013;**8**(4):e60788

[37] Kanai Y, Dohmae N, Hirokawa N. Kinesin transports RNA: Isolation and characterization of an RNA-transporting granule. Neuron. 2004;**43**(4):513-525

[38] Udagawa T, Fujioka Y, Tanaka M, Honda D, Yokoi S, Riku Y, et al. FUS regulates AMPA receptor function and FTLD/ALS-associated behaviour via GluA1 mRNA stabilization. Nature Communications. 2015;**6**:7098

[39] Tyzack GE, Luisier R, Taha DM, Neeves J, Modic M, Mitchell JS, et al. Widespread FUS mislocalization is a molecular hallmark of amyotrophic lateral sclerosis. Brain. 2019;**142**(9):2572-2580

[40] Bosco DA, Lemay N, Ko HK, Zhou H, Burke C, Kwiatkowski TJ Jr, et al. Mutant FUS proteins that cause amyotrophic lateral sclerosis incorporate into stress granules. Human Molecular Genetics. 2010;**19**(21):4160-4175

[41] Kamelgarn M, Chen J, Kuang L, Jin H, Kasarskis EJ, Zhu H. ALS mutations of FUS suppress protein translation and disrupt the regulation of nonsense-mediated decay. Proceedings of the National Academy of Sciences of the United States of America. 2018;**115**(51):E11904-E11913

[42] Yasuda K, Zhang H, Loiselle D, Haystead T, Macara IG, Mili S. The RNA-binding protein Fus directs translation of localized mRNAs in APC-RNP granules. The Journal of Cell Biology. 2013;**203**(5):737-746

[43] Marrone L, Drexler HCA, Wang J, Tripathi P, Distler T, Heisterkamp P, et al. FUS pathology in ALS is linked to alterations in multiple ALS-associated proteins and rescued by drugs stimulating autophagy. Acta Neuropathologica. 2019;**138**(1):67-84

[44] Kim GH, Kim JE, Rhie SJ, Yoon S. The role of oxidative stress in neurodegenerative diseases. Experimental Neurobiology. 2015;**24**(4):325-340

[45] De Luca G, Russo MT, Degan P, Tiveron C, Zijno A, Meccia E, et al. A role for oxidized DNA precursors in Huntington's disease-like striatal neurodegeneration. PLoS Genetics. 2008;**4**(11):e1000266

[46] Zhang J, Perry G, Smith MA, Robertson D, Olson SJ, Graham DG, et al. Parkinson's disease is associated with oxidative damage to cytoplasmic DNA and RNA in substantia nigra

neurons. The American Journal of Pathology. 1999;**154**(5):1423-1429

[47] Hegde ML, Hegde PM, Rao KS, Mitra S. Oxidative genome damage and its repair in neurodegenerative diseases: Function of transition metals as a double-edged sword. Journal of Alzheimer's Disease. 2011;**24**(Suppl 2): 183-198

[48] Castellotti B, Mariotti C, Rimoldi M, Fancellu R, Plumari M, Caimi S, et al. Ataxia with oculomotor apraxia type1 (AOA1): Novel and recurrent aprataxin mutations, coenzyme Q10 analyses, and clinical findings in Italian patients. Neurogenetics. 2011;**12**(3):193-201

[49] El-Khamisy SF, Saifi GM, Weinfeld M, Johansson F, Helleday T, Lupski JR, et al. Defective DNA single-strand break repair in spinocerebellar ataxia with axonal neuropathy-1. Nature. 2005;**434**(7029):108-113

[50] Wang H, Guo W, Mitra J, Hegde PM, Vandoorne T, Eckelmann BJ, et al. Mutant FUS causes DNA ligation defects to inhibit oxidative damage repair in amyotrophic lateral sclerosis. Nature Communications. 2018;**9**(1):3683

[51] Mastrocola AS, Kim SH, Trinh AT, Rodenkirch LA, Tibbetts RS. The RNA-binding protein fused in sarcoma (FUS) functions downstream of poly(ADP-ribose) polymerase (PARP) in response to DNA damage. The Journal of Biological Chemistry. 2013;**288**(34):24731-24741

[52] Rulten SL, Rotheray A, Green RL, Grundy GJ, Moore DA, Gomez-Herreros F, et al. PARP-1 dependent recruitment of the amyotrophic lateral sclerosis-associated protein FUS/TLS to sites of oxidative DNA damage. Nucleic Acids Research. 2014;**42**(1):307-314

[53] Altmeyer M, Neelsen KJ, Teloni F, Pozdnyakova I, Pellegrino S, Grofte M, et al. Liquid demixing of intrinsically disordered proteins is seeded by poly(ADP-ribose). Nature Communications. 2015;**6**:8088

[54] Greinert R, Volkmer B, Henning S, Breitbart EW, Greulich KO, Cardoso MC, et al. UVA-induced DNA double-strand breaks result from the repair of clustered oxidative DNA damages. Nucleic Acids Research. 2012;**40**(20):10263-10273

[55] Sallmann FR, Vodenicharov MD, Wang ZQ, Poirier GG. Characterization of sPARP-1. An alternative product of PARP-1 gene with poly(ADP-ribose) polymerase activity independent of DNA strand breaks. The Journal of Biological Chemistry. 2000;**275**(20):15504-15511

[56] Ko HL, Ren EC. Functional aspects of PARP1 in DNA repair and transcription. Biomolecules. 2012;**2**(4):524-548

[57] Shibata A, Kamada N, Masumura K, Nohmi T, Kobayashi S, Teraoka H, et al. Parp-1 deficiency causes an increase of deletion mutations and insertions/rearrangements in vivo after treatment with an alkylating agent. Oncogene. 2005;**24**(8):1328-1337

[58] Singatulina AS, Hamon L, Sukhanova MV, Desforges B, Joshi V, Bouhss A, et al. PARP-1 activation directs FUS to DNA damage sites to form PARG-reversible compartments enriched in damaged DNA. Cell Reports. 2019;**27**(6):1809-1821

[59] Patel A, Lee HO, Jawerth L, Maharana S, Jahnel M, Hein MY, et al. A liquid-to-solid phase transition of the ALS protein FUS accelerated by disease mutation. Cell. 2015;**162**(5):1066-1077

[60] Naumann M, Pal A, Goswami A, Lojewski X, Japtok J, Vehlow A, et al. Impaired DNA damage response signaling by FUS-NLS mutations

leads to neurodegeneration and FUS aggregate formation. Nature Communications. 2018;**9**(1):335

[61] Hoell JI, Larsson E, Runge S, Nusbaum JD, Duggimpudi S, Farazi TA, et al. RNA targets of wild-type and mutant FET family proteins. Nature Structural & Molecular Biology. 2011;**18**(12):1428-1431

[62] Zhou Y, Liu S, Liu G, Ozturk A, Hicks GG. ALS-associated FUS mutations result in compromised FUS alternative splicing and autoregulation. PLoS Genetics. 2013;**9**(10):e1003895

[63] Ishigaki S, Masuda A, Fujioka Y, Iguchi Y, Katsuno M, Shibata A, et al. Position-dependent FUS-RNA interactions regulate alternative splicing events and transcriptions. Scientific Reports. 2012;**2**:529

[64] Nakaya T, Alexiou P, Maragkakis M, Chang A, Mourelatos Z. FUS regulates genes coding for RNA-binding proteins in neurons by binding to their highly conserved introns. RNA. 2013;**19**(4):498-509

[65] Rogelj B, Easton LE, Bogu GK, Stanton LW, Rot G, Curk T, et al. Widespread binding of FUS along nascent RNA regulates alternative splicing in the brain. Scientific Reports. 2012;**2**:603

[66] Bradley WG, Krasin F. A new hypothesis of the etiology of amyotrophic lateral sclerosis. The DNA hypothesis. Archives of Neurology. 1982;**39**(11):677-680

[67] Madabhushi R, Gao F, Pfenning AR, Pan L, Yamakawa S, Seo J, et al. Activity-induced DNA breaks govern the expression of neuronal early-response genes. Cell. 2015;**161**(7):1592-1605

[68] Deng J, Yang M, Chen Y, Chen X, Liu J, Sun S, et al. FUS interacts with HSP60 to promote mitochondrial damage. PLoS Genetics. 2015;**11**(9):e1005357

[69] Deng J, Wang P, Chen X, Cheng H, Liu J, Fushimi K, et al. FUS interacts with ATP synthase beta subunit and induces mitochondrial unfolded protein response in cellular and animal models. Proceedings of the National Academy of Sciences of the United States of America. 2018;**115**(41):E9678-E9686

[70] Nakaya T, Maragkakis M. Amyotrophic lateral sclerosis associated FUS mutation shortens mitochondria and induces neurotoxicity. Scientific Reports. 2018;**8**(1):15575

[71] Kia A, McAvoy K, Krishnamurthy K, Trotti D, Pasinelli P. Astrocytes expressing ALS-linked mutant FUS induce motor neuron death through release of tumor necrosis factor-alpha. Glia. 2018;**66**(5):1016-1033

[72] Nagai M, Re DB, Nagata T, Chalazonitis A, Jessell TM, Wichterle H, et al. Astrocytes expressing ALS-linked mutated SOD1 release factors selectively toxic to motor neurons. Nature Neuroscience. 2007;**10**(5):615-622

[73] Ragagnin AMG, Shadfar S, Vidal M, Jamali MS, Atkin JD. Motor neuron susceptibility in ALS/FTD. Frontiers in Neuroscience. 2019;**13**:532

Chapter 3

Senataxin: A Putative RNA: DNA Helicase Mutated in ALS4—Emerging Mechanisms of Genome Stability in Motor Neurons

Arijit Dutta, Robert Hromas and Patrick Sung

Abstract

Amyotrophic lateral sclerosis type 4 (ALS4) is a rare, autosomal dominant childhood- or adolescent-onset motor neuron disease caused by genetic defects in senataxin (SETX), a putative RNA–DNA helicase. Studies on the yeast SETX ortholog Sen1 revealed its role in small RNA termination pathways. It has been postulated that ALS4-associated neuronal pathologies could stem from defects in RNA metabolism and altered gene expression. Importantly, SETX prevents the accumulation of R-loops, which are potentially pathogenic RNA–DNA hybrids that stem from perturbations in transcription. SETX also interacts with the tumor suppressor BRCA1 that helps promote DNA double-strand break repair by homologous recombination. As such, SETX could contribute toward the removal of harmful R-loops and DSBs in postmitotic neurons. This chapter will visit the plausible mechanistic role of SETX in R-loop removal and DNA break repair that could prevent the activation of apoptotic cell death in neurons and pathological manifestation of ALS4.

Keywords: spinal muscular atrophy, SETX, transcription, R-loop, DNA double-strand break, homologous recombination, nonhomologous DNA end joining

1. Introduction

Amyotrophic lateral sclerosis (ALS) type 4 is a rare form of distal spinal muscular atrophy (SMA) with onset at age 25 years or younger. The disease first manifests itself with weakness of ankles and wrists and gradually paralyzes the limbs due to severe muscle wasting. However, unlike classical ALS, the respiratory and bulbar muscles, sensory abilities, and cognitive functions are largely preserved in ALS4 patients. Hence, ALS4 patients, while having to endure severe disabilities, could expect an otherwise normal life expectancy with proper medical attention.

In 1998, the joint effort of Phillip Chance and David Cornblath described the Mattingly disease, a hereditary peripheral neuropathy as ALS type 4 (ALS4) [1]. The Mattingly disease was first seen among the descendants of a seventeenth-century English colonist, Thomas Mattingly from Maryland. With collaborations of the Mattingly clan, the work of Chance and Cornblath led to the identification of the disease gene locus located at chromosome 9q34 [1]. The causative gene was identified to be *Senataxin* (SETX), which is a large protein with features that typify RNA–DNA helicases [2]. Three distinct mutations in SETX were found in pedigree analysis of ALS4 patients. Some later studies also reported sporadic mutations in SETX [3, 4], which are summarized in **Table 1**. It should be noted that the other three forms of juvenile ALS (JALS) stem from mutations in different genes, namely, *ALS2* (ALS2), *SPG11* (ALS5), and *SIGMAR1* (ALS16).

Pathological studies of ALS4 have been hampered because of the rarity of the disease, with only about a dozen of diagnosed families around the world. Chen et al. [2] detected degeneration of anterior horn cells in spinal cords and cortico-spinal tracts in postmortem tissues from two aged individuals of pedigree K7000. Specifically, even though sensory abilities were not significantly affected in these individuals, a significant loss of dorsal root ganglia and posterior columns was detected, along with marked axonal degeneration of motor and sensory roots and peripheral nerves.

In another study, cytosolic mislocalization of the transactive response DNA-binding protein (TDP-43) was observed in spinal cord motor neurons in postmortem tissues from all the ALS4 patients examined [8]. TDP-43 is an RNA metabolism factor and is a well-documented biomarker that forms toxic protein aggregates in multiple neurodegenerative diseases including ALS [9, 10]. Recapitulation of TDP-43 histopathology in motor neurons of mice carrying ALS4 mutations led the authors to imply that dysfunction of SETX converges on TDP-43 pathology causing an ALS-type motor neurodegeneration [8], although the mechanism was not identified.

SETX has also been found mutated in another neurodegenerative disorder termed ataxia with oculomotor apraxia type 2 (AOA2) [11]. However, in this case, disease is caused by missense mutations leading to premature termination of the SETX mRNA transcript. AOA2 patients suffer from progressive cerebellar ataxia with peripheral neuropathy, cerebellar atrophy, and occasional oculomotor apraxia. However, unlike in ALS4, the motor neuron functions are largely preserved in AOA2 patients [12]. It has been suggested that distinct pathologies of AOA2 and ALS4 stem from unique alterations in expression of genes regulated via SETX in neuronal cells [13].

In spite of the seminal discovery of SETX mutations as being the root cause of ALS4, the etiopathogenesis of this disease remains largely unknown. In this

Mutation	Amino acid substitution	Family history	Origin	References
c.8C → T	T3I	Positive	Austria	Chen et al. [2]
c.1166T → C	L389S	Positive Positive	United States Italy	Rabin et al. [5] Chen et al. [2] Avemaria et al. [6]
c.2672T → T	V891A	Positive	Germany	Rudnik-Schoneborn et al. [7]
c.4660T → G	C1554G	Negative	United States	Hirano et al. [3]
c.6085C → G	K2029Q	Negative	United States	Hirano et al. [3]
c.6407G → A	R2136H	Positive	Belgium	Chen et al. 2004 [2]
c.6406C → T	R2136C	Negative	Japan	Saiga T et al., 2012 [4]
c.7640T → C	I2547T	Negative	United States	Hirano et al. [3]

Table 1.
ALS4-associated mutations in SETX.

chapter we will consider the properties of SETX and its role in the maintenance of genomic stability that are likely germane for the health of motor neurons and ALS4 pathology.

2. Senataxin at the crossroads of RNA metabolism and genomic stability

Studies on SETX predate its ALS4 association. SETX is the likely ortholog of a budding yeast protein, splicing endonuclease 1 (Sen1), so named because of its suspected role in the endonucleolytic processing of tRNA during its splicing and maturation [14]. However, because Sen1 lacks endonuclease activity, it likely functions as a non-catalytic effecter of the nucleolytic entity within the splicing machinery [15]. Sen1 possesses sequence motifs characteristic of superfamily 1 (SF1B) nucleic acid helicases [16]. Consistent with this, Sen1 possesses a helicase activity capable of unwinding RNA-DNA hybrids [17–19]. Like other SF1B helicases, Sen1 translocates on nucleic acid strands in the $5' \rightarrow 3'$ direction [20].

SETX is of low abundance (<500 molecules/cell) predominantly a nuclear protein with some studies reporting its presence in the nucleolus [21, 22]. SETX interacts with RNA polymerase II (pol II) and helps ensure correct termination of transcription and, as such, is important for the processing of noncoding RNAs (ncRNAs) and mRNAs [23, 24]. Importantly, recent studies suggest a role of SETX in maintaining genomic stability across highly transcribed genomic regions via resolution of RNA–DNA hybrids called R-loops, which arise as a consequence of RNA pol II stalling or perturbations of a transcription-coupled process such as mRNA splicing [25]. Moreover, SETX could also clear RNA–DNA hybrids at genomic breaks and promote DNA repair via homologous recombination (HR) [26]. We will explore the various functions of SETX/Sen1 and possible mechanisms by which SETX mutations give rise to ALS4.

2.1 Biochemical and structural features of SETX

SETX is a large protein of 2677 amino acid residues (303 kDa) and, like yeast Sen1, harbors SF1B-type helicase motifs (**Figure 1A**). It should be noted that even though Sen1 is known to unwind RNA-DNA hybrids [14, 15], such an activity has not yet been demonstrated for SETX. However, ALS4-associated missense mutations (K2029Q, R2136H, and I2547T) are all located in the putative C-terminal helicase domain of SETX (**Figure 1A**). Both SETX and Sen1 have an N-terminal domain that undergoes SUMO modification (**Figure 1A**) and that mediates protein–protein interactions with factors that function in RNA metabolism [27]. SETX likely forms a homodimer via the N-terminal domain, but the hereditary ALS4 mutations do not appear to affect protein dimerization [28].

2.1.1 SETX has a large intrinsically disordered region (IDR)

In silico analysis suggests that there is a large IDR in SETX that spans more than 1000 amino acid residues, a structural feature that is absent in the yeast ortholog Sen1. This putative IDR could confer to SETX the ability to interact with different protein partners, to bind nucleic acids [29]. IDRs in nucleic acid-binding proteins are often subject to post-translational modifications and could undergo phase separation, a molecular phenomenon of rearrangement of molecules in a homogenous solution into distinctly concentrated regions of space called condensates [30–33]. However, unrestrained phase separation causes protein aggregation that is observed with FUS [34] and TDP-43 [35], two extensively studied factors associated with

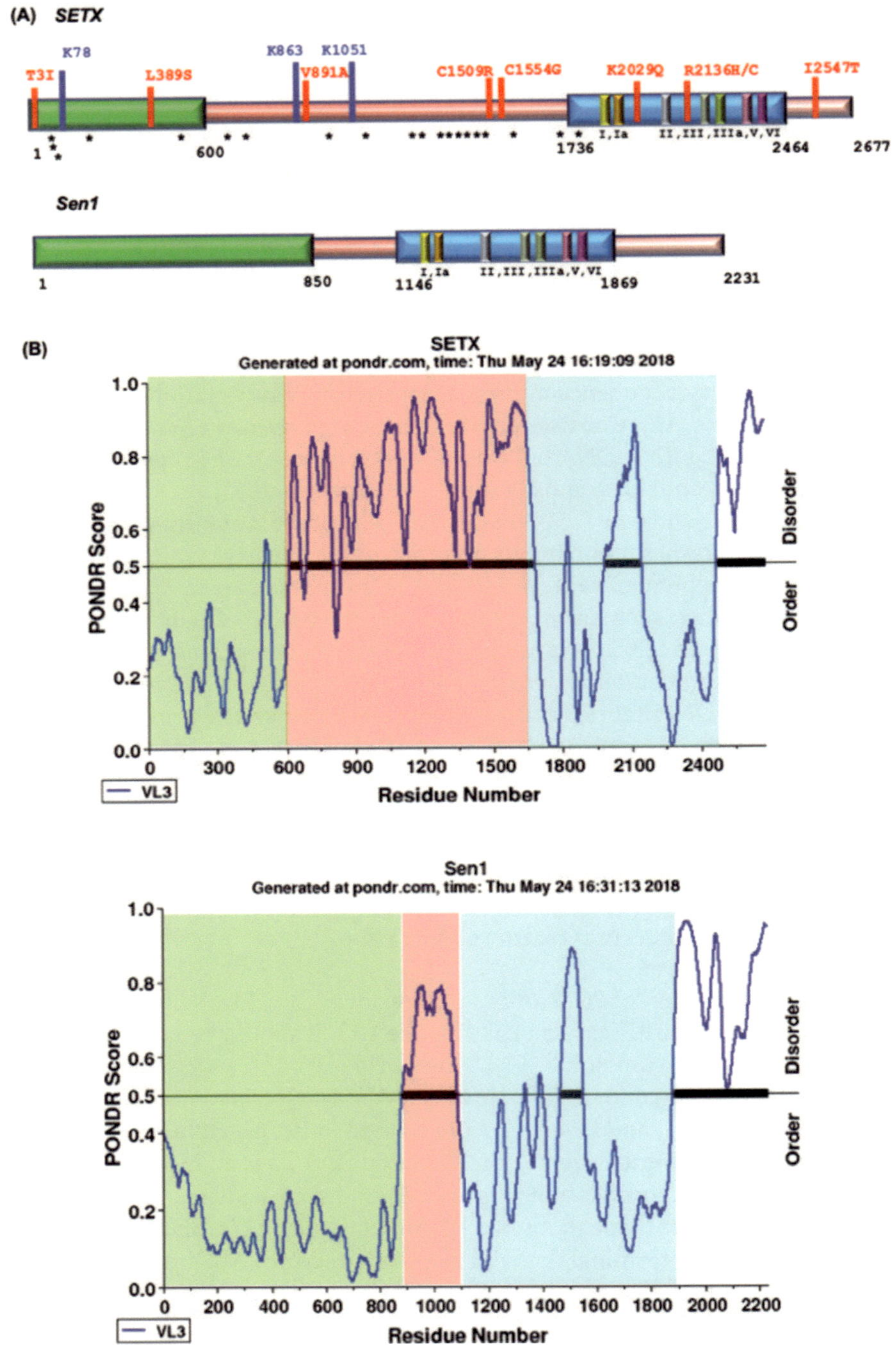

Figure 1.

(A) Schematic diagram of SETX, indicating N-terminal domain (green), central domain (red), and C-terminal helicase domain (blue); conserved motifs are highlighted: Motif I interacts with Mg2+ and NTP, conserved G maintains a flexible loop, motif 1a binds with substrate nucleic acid and transduces energy from the ATP-binding site to the DNA-binding site, motif II binds and hydrolyses ATP, motif III couples ATP hydrolysis with helicase activity, motif V binds substrate nucleic acid, and motif VI couples ATP hydrolysis with helicase activity; ALS4 mutation residues (red) are T3I, L389S, V891A, C1554G, K2029Q, R1236H/C, and I2647T; predicted sumoylation residues (blue) are K78, K863, and K1051 [119]; and cysteine residues predicted by CYSPRED (reliability≥8) to form disulfide bonds (indicated by stars) are C4, C5, C7, C145, C555, C637, C688, C997, C1080, C1123C,1153, C1262, C1277, C1398, C1442, C1509, C1672, C1719, and C2622. (B) Prediction of natural disordered region of SETX (upper panel), and Sen1 (lower panel), with the in silico metapredictor PONDR-VL3 [120]. N-terminal domain (green), central disordered region (red), C-terminal helicase domain (blue).

ALS, which are known to form stress granules in diseased neurons. It could be that SETX, through a phase separation mechanism, forms macromolecular complexes with factors associated with transcription and DNA damage repair. Pathological mutations in SETX could then lead to protein aggregation and loss of protein function in ALS4. This premise awaits experimental testing.

2.1.2 SETX structure could be regulated via disulfide bonding

Multiple neurodegenerative diseases including ALS have been classified among protein misfolding disorders, with disruption of protein disulfide isomerases (PDIs) causing aggregation of superoxide dismutase (SOD1) and TDP-43 in ALS neurons [36]. PDIs are a family of proteins that catalyze formation of disulfide bonds and proper folding of proteins, particularly especially those that harbor an IDR [37]. SETX has 31 cysteine residues in its IDR, and in silico analysis of this region using two independent neural network based predictors, CYSPRED [38] and DIpro [39], revealed that at least 14 cysteine residues in the SETX IDR could engage in disulfide bonding (**Figure 1A**), which is expected to be catalyzed by a PDI. This notion is supported by a proteomic analysis where PDIA6 was detected as a component of the SETX-interactome (**Figure 2**), [40]. We also note that amino acid residue C1554, expected to engage in disulfide linkage with C1509 (**Figure 1A**), is mutated in a sporadic case of ALS4 [3]. Testing of SETX regulation via redox homeostasis [41, 42] merits the effort of ALS researchers.

2.2 Involvement of SETX in RNA metabolism

2.2.1 Role in transcription termination

The role of SETX in regulation of coding and noncoding transcripts is highly conserved. RNA-seq analysis showed that SETX mutations that cause either ALS4 or AOA2 induce unique changes in gene expression patterns [13]. Studies in yeast have shown that Sen1 interacts directly with RNA pol II and is an integral component of the transcription termination machinery consisting of two other

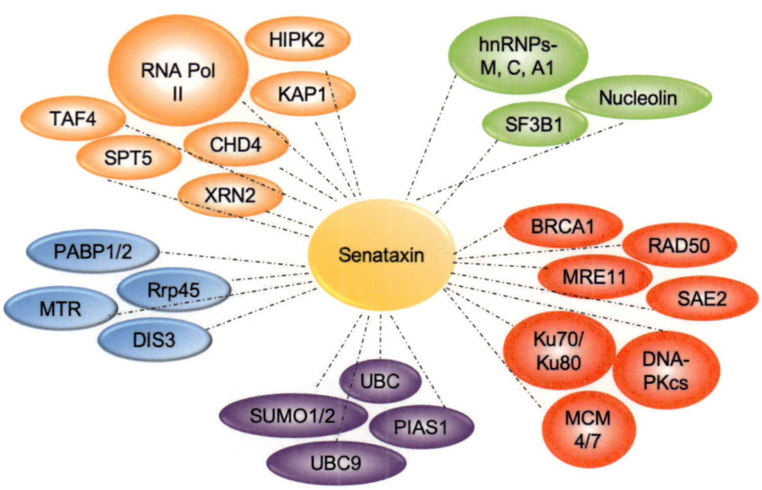

Figure 2.
SETX interactome: DNA repair factors (red), sumoylation and ubiquitination-associated factors (purple), RNA exosome factors (blue), RNAP II and transcription-associated factors (orange), splicing factor and RNA-binding proteins (green), adapted from [40].

factors (Nrd1 and Nab3) that regulate the generation of small nuclear RNAs (snRNAs) and small nucleolar RNAs (snoRNAs) [43–45]. During aberrant RNA pol II pausing, the Nrd1-Nab3-Sen1 (NNS) complex is recruited via direct interaction of Sen1 and Nrd1 with the C-terminal domain (CTD) of RNA pol II [46, 47]. Moreover, Pcf11, a component of the cleavage and polyadenylation complex (CPAC), facilitates RNA pol II CTD Ser2 phosphorylation and handoff of Sen1 from the NNS complex to RNA pol II [48]. NNS complex also captures polyadenylated RNAs and channels them to the RNA exosome complex for degradation, which we will discuss further in Section 2.2.2 [49]. Sen1 is also necessary for recruitment of Rat1/Xrn2, a 5′ → 3′ exoribonuclease at G-rich RNA pol II pause sites for degradation of the nascent transcripts and to prevent the accumulation of pathogenic R-loops [18, 50, 51]. Human lymphoblastoid and fibroblast cells with loss of both SETX or XRN2 result in increased R-loops and DNA double-strand breaks (DSBs) at transcriptional pause sites and hypersensitivity of cells to replications of stress and DNA damage induced by ionizing radiation, ultraviolet light, and oxidative stress [52, 53], which will be discussed further in Section 2.3.3. Thus, defects in pathways of RNA metabolism can lead to the induction of DNA damage.

2.2.2 Role in RNA surveillance machinery

SETX interacts with the RNA exosome, a highly conserved multiprotein ribonuclease complex that processes or degrades a diverse spectrum of RNAs in cells [54]. The exosome removes improperly processed coding and noncoding RNAs (ncRNAs) in the nucleus and regulates mRNA turnover in the cytoplasm. Other critical functions of the exosome include generation of mature ribosomal RNAs, processing of ncRNAs into snRNAs and snoRNAs, and turnover of tRNAs. The human RNA exosome is a ten-subunit complex with a central six-subunit core that constitutes a channel (EXOSC4–9), a three-subunit cap (EXOSC1–3) and a ribonuclease (EXOSC11) subunit located at the bottom of the channel. The nuclear form of the exosome also harbors a riboexonuclease subunit, EXOSC10 [54, 55]. The current model posits that a RNA strand enters the exosome through the cap and is threaded through the channel to be fed to the ribonuclease module for nucleolytic processing [55].

Importantly, SETX interacts with EXOSC9, and complex formation requires SUMOylation of the N-terminal domain of SETX [27]. It has been inferred that SETX-exosome interaction reflects a vital mechanistic axis for resolving co-transcriptional R-loops and preventing genomic instability at heavily transcribed regions in neurons. It might also be surmised that the RNA exosome is recruited via SETX at R-loops to help resolve these pathogenic structures via degradation of the RNA moiety.

Interestingly, the RNA exosome has also been linked to spinal SMA-type neuropathies. Familial missense mutations in EXOSC3 [56] and EXOSC8 [57] are linked to an infantile neuronal disorder, pontocerebellar hypoplasia type 1 (PCH1), that is marked by cerebellar atrophy and progressive microcephaly along with developmental defects and degeneration of spinal motor neurons. Hereditary mutations in EXOSC10 also cause similar neurological defects [58]. Taken together, the available evidence points to a critical role of the exosome in the avoidance of motor neuropathies. Given the interaction noted for SETX and exosome, it might be contemplated that an R-loop removal defect in spinal motor neuronal precursor and differentiated cells could represent the underlying basis for PCH1.

2.3 SETX: a guardian of genomic stability across highly transcribed genomic landscapes

2.3.1 Transcription-coupled (TC) repair

Nucleotide excision repair (NER) is a conserved DNA repair pathway that removes bulky DNA lesions such as those induced by ultraviolet light. When the RNA polymerase II ensemble is obstructed by such a bulky lesion, Cockayne syndrome B (CSB) protein, which interacts with RNA pol II, mediates the recruitment of NER factors such as the Cockayne syndrome A (CSA)-E3-ubiquitin ligase complex [59] and the endonucleases ERCC1-XPF and XPG to mediate the removal of the DNA lesion. In yeast cells, Sen1 has been shown to play a direct role in TC-NER via interaction with Rad2, the yeast XPG ortholog [47]. Whether SETX also functions in TC-NER in humans remains an open question. However, in the absence of SETX, the TC-NER endonucleases XPF and XPG generate DSBs at R-loops, leading to the activation of DNA damage response pathways and repair via HR or the alternate DSB repair pathway of nonhomologous DNA end joining (NHEJ) [60].

2.3.2 Resolution of R-loops

R-loops are RNA–DNA hybrid structures with a displaced single DNA strand and are generated upon reannealing of a nascent transcript with the sense strand [61]. R-loops are transiently formed in many regions of the genome, including those transcribed by RNA pol I, II, and III [62]. R-loops are abundant at promoters of RNA pol II-transcribed genes [63–65], at sequences that are prone to forming G-quadruplex or hairpin structures in the non-template DNA strand [66]. Perturbations of transcription-coupled processes, such as mRNA splicing, also result in R-loop formation [61, 67]. R-loops are detected in the genome via DNA–RNA immunoprecipitation (DRIP) [68] and immunofluorescence assays with the monoclonal antibody S9.6, which has high affinity for RNA–DNA hybrids [69]. Typically, to ensure that the signal detected is specific for RNA–DNA hybrids, one would include the expression of RNase H in cells (to digest the hybrids) or pretreat samples for sequencing with this enzyme.

Depending upon their location and size, R-loops could impart beneficial or harmful effects. R-loops could extend from a few hundred base pairs to kilo base pairs in size. In immunoglobulin (Ig) class switch regions, R-loops serve an important role in Ig class switch recombination by promoting the induction of DNA breaks via the action of activation-induced cytidine deaminase (AID) and base excision repair factors [70]. R-loops also prime DNA replication in the mitochondrial genome [71]. In human fibroblast cells, R-loops can influence the expression of over 1200 genes by facilitating transcription via suppression of DNA methylation [72] and recruitment or eviction of chromatin remodeling complexes [73]. On the contrary, R-loops could interfere with transcription at certain genomic loci like rDNA [62, 74]. The major threat from unscheduled R-loops is the generation of lethal DSBs because of head-on collisions with the DNA replication machinery [75, 76].

Because of the potential harm that R-loops could cause, their levels are tightly regulated via a variety of mechanisms. In this regard, RNAseH1/2 provides a major means for R-loop clearance via ribonucleolytic cleavage of RNA strand [77, 78]. While topoisomerase I prevents R-loop formation by reducing negative supercoiling behind the elongating RNA pol II, TRanscription EXport (TREX) complex factors (THOC1–7, UAP56) and serine–/arginine-rich splicing factor 1 (SRSF1) suppress R-loops by removing the nascent mRNA [79]. RNA biogenesis factors like Trf4/Air2/Mtr4p polyadenylation

(TRAMP) complex and, as discussed earlier, the RNA exosome complex also participate in the regulation of R-loop formation or removal [80]. Moreover, R-loops can be dissociated via the nucleic acid unwinding activity of Sen1/SETX [23, 50, 81] and other helicase proteins such as Pif1 [82], DEAH box protein 9 (DHX9) [83], and Fanconi Anemia Complementation factor M (FANCM) [84]. It seems reasonable to postulate that each of the above-named factors operates at specific genomic milieu.

Studies so forth have suggested that SETX is involved in resolving R-loops at paused transcription sites [50] via forming a physiological complex with the tumor suppressor protein BRCA1 to prevent R-loop-associated DNA damage [25]. This warrants further investigation on SETX-BRCA1 axis to reveal the molecular mechanisms of R-loop resolution.

2.3.3 DNA double-strand break repair and replication fork stability

Occurrence of DSBs and their repair in terminally differentiated neurons were reported in the early 1970s [85, 86]. Recent studies have provided evidence that ALS is associated with a defect in DSB repair [87–89]. DSBs are generated in neurons via endogenous oxidative stress [90, 91] or a topoisomerase IIβ-dependent mechanism that is essential for expression of early genes regulating vital neuronal functions [92]. A recent study showed that neuronal cells from SMA express only low levels of SETX and DNA-PKcs, a highly conserved NHEJ factor. As a result, SMA neurons display higher levels of R-loops that culminate DSB formation, and cellular toxicity [93]. Importantly, these phenotypic manifestations can be corrected by the overexpression of SETX. These observations aptly underscore the genome protective role of SETX in neurons.

Importantly, SETX colocalizes at DSBs with various factors that function in the DNA damage response and repair factors, including γH2AX, 53BP1, and BRCA1, and it forms a co-immunoprecipitable complex with DNA-PKcs, MRE11, RAD50 [24, 25, 53, 94]. AOA2-pateint derived lymphoblastoid cell lines lacking SETX are sensitive toward topoisomerase I inhibitor, camptothecin, DNA crosslinking agent mitomycin C and hydrogen peroxide [53], again indicative of a role of SETX in the DNA damage response. Moreover, *Setx−/−* mice displays a defect in germ cell maturation due to defective meiotic recombination with unrepaired DSBs [81]. Interestingly, recent findings revealed that nascent transcripts or small ncRNAs could accumulate at DSBs via diverse mechanisms, and affect DSB repair via distinct pathways of HR or NHEJ [95–103]. This was further evidenced by the studies demonstrating that both excess removal and impaired clearance of RNA–DNA hybrids result in defective DSB repair [100], suggesting the role of RNA in DSB repair via processes that are yet to be characterized. In this context, SETX has been implicated in enhancing HR-mediated DSB repair that is catalyzed by the recombinase RAD51, via resolving RNA–DNA hybrids at DSBs [26]. Further biochemical investigations are required to dissect the mechanistic underpinnings of this process.

It should be noted that cycling cells face an incessant threat of genomic instability via replication-transcription collisions, wherein the replication and transcription machineries could engage in head-on collisions [104]. This could directly lead to formation of DSBs [76]. Importantly, SETX associates with DNA replication forks and promotes their progression across RNA pol II transcribed regions, a function that appears to be independent of its transcription termination role [105].

2.3.4 Telomere maintenance

Telomeres, which comprise repetitive DNA sequences, cap the ends of each chromosome, and their attrition leads to cellular senescence. Telomerase reverse transcriptase (TERT), the catalytic subunit of telomerase that maintains the normal length of telomeres, is present at a low level in most differentiated cells including neurons [106]. TERT levels appear to be significantly lower in the spinal cord tissues of ALS patients than healthy individuals [107]. Ex vivo studies have suggested that while telomere damage induces neuronal cell death [108], the activation of telomerase can enhance neuronal cell viability [109, 110]. Interestingly, a novel compound that enhances telomerase activity in neurons also appears to ameliorate the symptoms of ALS [109].

Importantly, SETX is present at telomeres, and AOA2 lymphocytes and lymphoblasts showed reduced telomere length along with higher sensitivity toward oxidative stress and DNA-damaging agents [111]. Another study has implicated SETX in the maintenance of telomeres in *Myotis* bats [112]. These observations should constitute the basis for investigating the mechanistic role of SETX in telomere maintenance in motor neurons and other cell types.

3. Conclusion

Defects in RNA metabolism factors have been associated with multiple motor neuron diseases including ALS and SMA [113, 114]. Despite having distinctive pathological manifestations and clinical onsets, such motor neuropathies could stem from related underlying mechanisms pertaining to RNA homeostasis. In this chapter, we reviewed how defective RNA metabolic pathways could ensue genomic instability, an emerging mechanism in neurodegenerative diseases. Co-transcriptional R-loops are crucial for regulating gene expression in both dividing and postmitotic neurons; however, when not timely resolved, it will lead to genomic instability via generation of DNA strand breaks. While replication-transcription conflicts are the major source of R-loop-induced DSBs in dividing cells that need repair via HR or NHEJ, how R-loops trigger DSBs in postmitotic neurons remains to be investigated. Moreover, small RNAs at DSBs could impede repair and must be cleared nucleolytically or via unwinding of RNA–DNA hybrids. Genetic and cell-based studies of human SETX, together with biochemical characterization of its yeast ortholog Sen1, have suggested that SETX protects genomic stability via resolution of R-loops, assisting replication fork progression across transcribing genomic regions and promoting HR at DSBs. In the light of recent findings on implication of genomic instability in neurodegenerative diseases, as reviewed in [115–118], in-depth studies are required to precisely delineate role of SETX in ALS4. Thus, it is apposite to test if ALS4 gain-of-function mutations affect SETX activities pertaining to DSB repair.

Treatment of ALS4 or other JALS is currently limited to physical and occupational therapies to promote mobility and independence. While an FDA-approved glutamate inhibitor drug, riluzole, that slows down symptoms and prolongs survival is used clinically to treat ALS, there are currently no specific treatment for juvenile ALS diseases. Further studies are obligatory to recognize SETX as a therapeutic target for treatment of ALS4.

Acknowledgements

Dr. Dutta has been supported by a Brown-Coxe postdoctoral fellowship from Yale University School of Medicine and a Jeane B. Kempner postdoctoral fellowship from the University of Texas Medical Branch, Galveston. The laboratories of Robert Hromas and Patrick Sung have been funded by research grants from the US

National Institutes of Health. Patrick Sung is a CPRIT Scholar in Cancer Research and the holder of the Robert A. Welch Distinguished Chair in Chemistry.

Conflict of interest

The authors declare no conflict of interest.

Author details

Arijit Dutta[1], Robert Hromas[2] and Patrick Sung[1*]

1 Department of Biochemistry and Structural Biology, University of Texas Health Science Center at San Antonio, San Antonio, TX, USA

2 Department of Medicine, University of Texas Health Science Center at San Antonio, San Antonio, TX, USA

*Address all correspondence to: sungp@uthscsa.edu

References

[1] Chance PF, Rabin BA, Ryan SG, Ding Y, Scavina M, Crain B, et al. Linkage of the gene for an autosomal dominant form of juvenile amyotrophic lateral sclerosis to chromosome 9q34. American Journal of Human Genetics. 1998;**62**:633-640

[2] Chen YZ, Bennett CL, Huynh HM, Blair IP, Puls I, Irobi J, et al. DNA/RNA helicase gene mutations in a form of juvenile amyotrophic lateral sclerosis (ALS4). American Journal of Human Genetics. 2004;**74**:1128-1135

[3] Hirano M, Quinzii CM, Mitsumoto H, Hays AP, Roberts JK, Richard P, et al. Senataxin mutations and amyotrophic lateral sclerosis. Amyotrophic Lateral Sclerosis. 2011;**12**:223-227

[4] Saiga T, Tateishi T, Torii T, Kawamura N, Nagara Y, Shigeto H, et al. Inflammatory radiculoneuropathy in an ALS4 patient with a novel SETX mutation. Journal of Neurology, Neurosurgery, and Psychiatry. 2012;**83**:763-764

[5] Rabin BA, Griffin JW, Crain BJ, Scavina M, Chance PF, Cornblath DR. Autosomal dominant juvenile amyotrophic lateral sclerosis. Brain. 1999;**122(Pt 8)**:1539-1550

[6] Avemaria F, Lunetta C, Tarlarini C, Mosca L, Maestri E, Marocchi A, et al. Mutation in the senataxin gene found in a patient affected by familial ALS with juvenile onset and slow progression. Amyotrophic Lateral Sclerosis. 2011;**12**:228-230

[7] Rudnik-Schoneborn S, Arning L, Epplen JT, Zerres K. SETX gene mutation in a family diagnosed autosomal dominant proximal spinal muscular atrophy. Neuromuscular Disorders. 2012;**22**:258-262

[8] Bennett CL, Dastidar SG, Ling SC, Malik B, Ashe T, Wadhwa M, et al. Senataxin mutations elicit motor neuron degeneration phenotypes and yield TDP-43 mislocalization in ALS4 mice and human patients. Acta Neuropathologica. 2018;**136**:425-443

[9] Gao J, Wang L, Huntley ML, Perry G, Wang X. Pathomechanisms of TDP-43 in neurodegeneration. Journal of Neurochemistry. 2018;**146**:7-20

[10] Cohen TJ, Lee VM, Trojanowski JQ. TDP-43 functions and pathogenic mechanisms implicated in TDP-43 proteinopathies. Trends in Molecular Medicine. 2011;**17**:659-667

[11] Moreira MC, Klur S, Watanabe M, Nemeth AH, Le Ber I, Moniz JC, et al. Senataxin, the ortholog of a yeast RNA helicase, is mutant in ataxia-ocular apraxia 2. Nature Genetics. 2004;**36**:225-227

[12] Anheim M, Monga B, Fleury M, Charles P, Barbot C, Salih M, et al. Ataxia with oculomotor apraxia type 2: Clinical, biological and genotype/phenotype correlation study of a cohort of 90 patients. Brain. 2009;**132**:2688-2698

[13] Fogel BL, Cho E, Wahnich A, Gao F, Becherel OJ, Wang X, et al. Mutation of senataxin alters disease-specific transcriptional networks in patients with ataxia with oculomotor apraxia type 2. Human Molecular Genetics. 2014;**23**:4758-4769

[14] Winey M, Culbertson MR. Mutations affecting the tRNA-splicing endonuclease activity of Saccharomyces cerevisiae. Genetics. 1988;**118**:609-617

[15] DeMarini DJ, Winey M, Ursic D, Webb F, Culbertson MR. SEN1, a positive effector of tRNA-splicing endonuclease in *Saccharomyces cerevisiae*.

Molecular and Cellular Biology. 1992;**12**:2154-2164

[16] Kim HD, Choe J, Seo YS. The sen1(+) gene of Schizosaccharomyces pombe, a homologue of budding yeast SEN1, encodes an RNA and DNA helicase. Biochemistry. 1999;**38**:14697-14710

[17] Martin-Tumasz S, Brow DA. Saccharomyces cerevisiae Sen1 helicase domain exhibits 5′- to 3'-helicase activity with a preference for translocation on DNA rather than RNA. The Journal of Biological Chemistry. 2015;**290**:22880-22889

[18] Han Z, Libri D, Porrua O. Biochemical characterization of the helicase Sen1 provides new insights into the mechanisms of non-coding transcription termination. Nucleic Acids Research. 2017;**45**:1355-1370

[19] Leonaite B, Han Z, Basquin J, Bonneau F, Libri D, Porrua O, et al. Sen1 has unique structural features grafted on the architecture of the Upf1-like helicase family. The EMBO Journal. 2017;**36**:1590-1604

[20] Buttner K, Nehring S, Hopfner KP. Structural basis for DNA duplex separation by a superfamily-2 helicase. Nature Structural & Molecular Biology. 2007;**14**:647-652

[21] Chen YZ, Hashemi SH, Anderson SK, Huang Y, Moreira MC, Lynch DR, et al. Senataxin, the yeast Sen1p orthologue: Characterization of a unique protein in which recessive mutations cause ataxia and dominant mutations cause motor neuron disease. Neurobiology of Disease. 2006;**23**:97-108

[22] Beck M, Schmidt A, Malmstroem J, Claassen M, Ori A, Szymborska A, et al. The quantitative proteome of a human cell line. Molecular Systems Biology. 2011;7:549

[23] Suraweera A, Lim Y, Woods R, Birrell GW, Nasim T, Becherel OJ, et al. Functional role for senataxin, defective in ataxia oculomotor apraxia type 2, in transcriptional regulation. Human Molecular Genetics. 2009;**18**:3384-3396

[24] Yuce O, West SC. Senataxin, defective in the neurodegenerative disorder ataxia with oculomotor apraxia 2, lies at the interface of transcription and the DNA damage response. Molecular and Cellular Biology. 2013;**33**:406-417

[25] Hatchi E, Skourti-Stathaki K, Ventz S, Pinello L, Yen A, Kamieniarz-Gdula K, et al. BRCA1 recruitment to transcriptional pause sites is required for R-loop-driven DNA damage repair. Molecular Cell. 2015;**57**:636-647

[26] Cohen S, Puget N, Lin YL, Clouaire T, Aguirrebengoa M, Rocher V, et al. Senataxin resolves RNA: DNA hybrids forming at DNA double-strand breaks to prevent translocations. Nature Communications. 2018;**9**:533

[27] Richard P, Feng S, Manley JL. A SUMO-dependent interaction between Senataxin and the exosome, disrupted in the neurodegenerative disease AOA2, targets the exosome to sites of transcription-induced DNA damage. Genes & Development. 2013;**27**:2227-2232

[28] Bennett CL, Chen Y, Vignali M, Lo RS, Mason AG, Unal A, et al. Protein interaction analysis of senataxin and the ALS4 L389S mutant yields insights into senataxin post-translational modification and uncovers mutant-specific binding with a brain cytoplasmic RNA-encoded peptide. PLoS One. 2013;**8**:e78837

[29] Oldfield CJ, Dunker AK. Intrinsically disordered proteins and intrinsically disordered protein regions.

Annual Review of Biochemistry. 2014;**83**:553-584

[30] Posey AE, Holehouse AS, Pappu RV. Phase separation of intrinsically disordered proteins. Methods in Enzymology. 2018;**611**:1-30

[31] Hahn S. Phase separation, protein disorder, and enhancer function. Cell. 2018;**175**:1723-1725

[32] Elbaum-Garfinkle S. Matter over mind: Liquid phase separation and neurodegeneration. The Journal of Biological Chemistry. 2019;**294**:7160-7168

[33] Boeynaems S, Alberti S, Fawzi NL, Mittag T, Polymenidou M, Rousseau F, et al. Protein phase separation: A new phase in cell biology. Trends in Cell Biology. 2018;**28**:420-435

[34] Patel A, Lee HO, Jawerth L, Maharana S, Jahnel M, Hein MY, et al. A liquid-to-solid phase transition of the ALS protein FUS accelerated by disease mutation. Cell. 2015;**162**:1066-1077

[35] Mann JR, Gleixner AM, Mauna JC, Gomes E, DeChellis-Marks MR, Needham PG, et al. RNA binding antagonizes neurotoxic phase transitions of TDP-43. Neuron. 2019;**102**:321-338

[36] Andreu CI, Woehlbier U, Torres M, Hetz C. Protein disulfide isomerases in neurodegeneration: From disease mechanisms to biomedical applications. FEBS Letters. 2012;**586**:2826-2834

[37] Hatahet F, Ruddock LW. Protein disulfide isomerase: A critical evaluation of its function in disulfide bond formation. Antioxidants & Redox Signaling. 2009;**11**:2807-2850

[38] Fariselli P, Riccobelli P, Casadio R. Role of evolutionary information in predicting the disulfide-bonding state of cysteine in proteins. Proteins. 1999;**36**:340-346

[39] Cheng J, Saigo H, Baldi P. Large-scale prediction of disulphide bridges using kernel methods, two-dimensional recursive neural networks, and weighted graph matching. Proteins. 2006;**62**:617-629

[40] Groh M, Albulescu LO, Cristini A, Gromak N. Senataxin: genome guardian at the interface of transcription and neurodegeneration. Journal of Molecular Biology. 2017;**429**:3181-3195

[41] Paul BD, Sbodio JI, Snyder SH. Cysteine metabolism in neuronal redox homeostasis. Trends in Pharmacological Sciences. 2018;**39**:513-524

[42] Franco R, Vargas MR. Redox biology in neurological function, dysfunction, and aging. Antioxidants & Redox Signaling. 2018;**28**:1583-1586

[43] Steinmetz EJ, Brow DA. Repression of gene expression by an exogenous sequence element acting in concert with a heterogeneous nuclear ribonucleoprotein-like protein, Nrd1, and the putative helicase Sen1. Molecular and Cellular Biology. 1996;**16**:6993-7003

[44] Steinmetz EJ, Conrad NK, Brow DA, Corden JL. RNA-binding protein Nrd1 directs poly(A)-independent 3′-end formation of RNA polymerase II transcripts. Nature. 2001;**413**:327-331

[45] Steinmetz EJ, Warren CL, Kuehner JN, Panbehi B, Ansari AZ, Brow DA. Genome-wide distribution of yeast RNA polymerase II and its control by Sen1 helicase. Molecular Cell. 2006;**24**:735-746

[46] Chinchilla K, Rodriguez-Molina JB, Ursic D, Finkel JS, Ansari AZ, Culbertson MR. Interactions of Sen1, Nrd1, and Nab3 with multiple phosphorylated forms of the Rpb1

C-terminal domain in Saccharomyces cerevisiae. Eukaryotic Cell. 2012;**11**:417-429

[47] Ursic D, Chinchilla K, Finkel JS, Culbertson MR. Multiple protein/protein and protein/RNA interactions suggest roles for yeast DNA/RNA helicase Sen1p in transcription, transcription-coupled DNA repair and RNA processing. Nucleic Acids Research. 2004;**32**:2441-2452

[48] Grzechnik P, Gdula MR, Proudfoot NJ. Pcf11 orchestrates transcription termination pathways in yeast. Genes & Development. 2015;**29**:849-861

[49] Arndt KM, Reines D. Termination of transcription of short noncoding RNAs by RNA polymerase II. Annual Review of Biochemistry. 2015;**84**:381-404

[50] Skourti-Stathaki K, Proudfoot NJ, Gromak N. Human senataxin resolves RNA/DNA hybrids formed at transcriptional pause sites to promote Xrn2-dependent termination. Molecular Cell. 2011;**42**:794-805

[51] Wagschal A, Rousset E, Basavarajaiah P, Contreras X, Harwig A, Laurent-Chabalier S, et al. Microprocessor, Setx, Xrn2, and Rrp6 co-operate to induce premature termination of transcription by RNAPII. Cell. 2012;**150**:1147-1157

[52] Morales JC, Richard P, Patidar PL, Motea EA, Dang TT, Manley JL, et al. XRN2 links transcription termination to DNA damage and replication stress. PLoS Genetics. 2016;**12**:e1006107

[53] Suraweera A, Becherel OJ, Chen P, Rundle N, Woods R, Nakamura J, et al. Senataxin, defective in ataxia oculomotor apraxia type 2, is involved in the defense against oxidative DNA damage. The Journal of Cell Biology. 2007;**177**:969-979

[54] Morton DJ, Kuiper EG, Jones SK, Leung SW, Corbett AH, Fasken MB. The RNA exosome and RNA exosome-linked disease. RNA. 2018;**24**:127-142

[55] Kilchert C, Wittmann S, Vasiljeva L. The regulation and functions of the nuclear RNA exosome complex. Nature Reviews. Molecular Cell Biology. 2016;**17**:227-239

[56] Wan J, Yourshaw M, Mamsa H, Rudnik-Schoneborn S, Menezes MP, Hong JE, et al. Mutations in the RNA exosome component gene EXOSC3 cause pontocerebellar hypoplasia and spinal motor neuron degeneration. Nature Genetics. 2012;**44**:704-708

[57] Boczonadi V, Muller JS, Pyle A, Munkley J, Dor T, Quartararo J, et al. EXOSC8 mutations alter mRNA metabolism and cause hypomyelination with spinal muscular atrophy and cerebellar hypoplasia. Nature Communications. 2014;**5**:4287

[58] Burns DT, Donkervoort S, Muller JS, Knierim E, Bharucha-Goebel D, Faqeih EA, et al. Variants in EXOSC9 disrupt the RNA exosome and result in cerebellar atrophy with spinal motor neuronopathy. American Journal of Human Genetics. 2018;**102**:858-873

[59] Fousteri M, Mullenders LH. Transcription-coupled nucleotide excision repair in mammalian cells: Molecular mechanisms and biological effects. Cell Research. 2008;**18**:73-84

[60] Sollier J, Stork CT, Garcia-Rubio ML, Paulsen RD, Aguilera A, Cimprich KA. Transcription-coupled nucleotide excision repair factors promote R-loop-induced genome instability. Molecular Cell. 2014;**56**:777-785

[61] Crossley MP, Bocek M, Cimprich KA. R-loops as cellular regulators and genomic threats. Molecular Cell. 2019;**73**:398-411

[62] El Hage A, French SL, Beyer AL, Tollervey D. Loss of topoisomerase I leads to R-loop-mediated transcriptional blocks during ribosomal RNA synthesis. Genes & Development. 2010;**24**:1546-1558

[63] Chen L, Chen JY, Zhang X, Gu Y, Xiao R, Shao C, et al. R-ChIP using inactive RNase H reveals dynamic coupling of R-loops with transcriptional pausing at gene promoters. Molecular Cell. 2017;**68**:745-757

[64] Ginno PA, Lott PL, Christensen HC, Korf I, Chedin F. R-loop formation is a distinctive characteristic of unmethylated human CpG island promoters. Molecular Cell. 2012;**45**:814-825

[65] Dumelie JG, Jaffrey SR. Defining the location of promoter-associated R-loops at near-nucleotide resolution using bisDRIP-seq. Elife. 2017;**6**:e28306

[66] Skourti-Stathaki K, Proudfoot NJ. A double-edged sword: R loops as threats to genome integrity and powerful regulators of gene expression. Genes & Development. 2014;**28**:1384-1396

[67] Li X, Manley JL. Inactivation of the SR protein splicing factor ASF/SF2 results in genomic instability. Cell. 2005;**122**:365-378

[68] Sanz LA, Chedin F. High-resolution, strand-specific R-loop mapping via S9.6-based DNA-RNA immunoprecipitation and high-throughput sequencing. Nature Protocols. 2019;**14**:1734-1755

[69] Boguslawski SJ, Smith DE, Michalak MA, Mickelson KE, Yehle CO, Patterson WL, et al. Characterization of monoclonal antibody to DNA.RNA and its application to immunodetection of hybrids. Journal of Immunological Methods. 1986;**89**:123-130

[70] Roy D, Yu K, Lieber MR. Mechanism of R-loop formation at immunoglobulin class switch sequences. Molecular and Cellular Biology. 2008;**28**:50-60

[71] Lee DY, Clayton DA. Initiation of mitochondrial DNA replication by transcription and R-loop processing. The Journal of Biological Chemistry. 1998;**273**:30614-30621

[72] Grunseich C, Wang IX, Watts JA, Burdick JT, Guber RD, Zhu Z, et al. Senataxin mutation reveals how R-loops promote transcription by blocking DNA methylation at gene promoters. Molecular Cell. 2018;**69**:426-437

[73] Chen PB, Chen HV, Acharya D, Rando OJ, Fazzio TG. R loops regulate promoter-proximal chromatin architecture and cellular differentiation. Nature Structural & Molecular Biology. 2015;**22**:999-1007

[74] Belotserkovskii BP, Soo Shin JH, Hanawalt PC. Strong transcription blockage mediated by R-loop formation within a G-rich homopurine-homopyrimidine sequence localized in the vicinity of the promoter. Nucleic Acids Research. 2017;**45**:6589-6599

[75] Gan W, Guan Z, Liu J, Gui T, Shen K, Manley JL, et al. R-loop-mediated genomic instability is caused by impairment of replication fork progression. Genes & Development. 2011;**25**:2041-2056

[76] Hamperl S, Bocek MJ, Saldivar JC, Swigut T, Cimprich KA. Transcription-replication conflict orientation modulates R-loop levels and activates distinct DNA damage responses. Cell. 2017;**170**:774-786

[77] El Hage A, Webb S, Kerr A, Tollervey D. Genome-wide distribution of RNA-DNA hybrids identifies RNase H targets in tRNA genes, retrotransposons and mitochondria. PLoS Genetics. 2014;**10**:e1004716

[78] Wahba L, Amon JD, Koshland D, Vuica-Ross M. RNase H and multiple

RNA biogenesis factors cooperate to prevent RNA:DNA hybrids from generating genome instability. Molecular Cell. 2011;**44**:978-988

[79] Santos-Pereira JM, Aguilera A. R loops: New modulators of genome dynamics and function. Nature Reviews. Genetics. 2015;**16**:583-597

[80] Laffleur B, Basu U. Biology of RNA surveillance in development and disease. Trends in Cell Biology. 2019;**29**:428-445

[81] Becherel OJ, Yeo AJ, Stellati A, Heng EY, Luff J, Suraweera AM, et al. Senataxin plays an essential role with DNA damage response proteins in meiotic recombination and gene silencing. PLoS Genetics. 2013;**9**:e1003435

[82] Tran PLT, Pohl TJ, Chen CF, Chan A, Pott S, Zakian VA. PIF1 family DNA helicases suppress R-loop mediated genome instability at tRNA genes. Nature Communications. 2017;**8**:15025

[83] Cristini A, Groh M, Kristiansen MS, Gromak N. RNA/DNA hybrid Interactome identifies DXH9 as a molecular player in transcriptional termination and R-loop-associated DNA damage. Cell Reports. 2018;**23**:1891-1905

[84] Schwab RA, Nieminuszczy J, Shah F, Langton J, Lopez Martinez D, Liang CC, et al. The fanconi anemia pathway maintains genome stability by coordinating replication and transcription. Molecular Cell. 2015;**60**:351-361

[85] Price GB, Modak SP, Makinodan T. Age-associated changes in the DNA of mouse tissue. Science. 1971;**171**:917-920

[86] Wheeler KT, Lett JT. Formation and rejoining of DNA strand breaks in irradiated neurons: in vivo. Radiation Research. 1972;**52**:59-67

[87] Mitra J, Guerrero EN, Hegde PM, Liachko NF, Wang H, Vasquez V, et al. Motor neuron disease-associated loss of nuclear TDP-43 is linked to DNA double-strand break repair defects. Proceedings of the National Academy of Sciences of the United States of America. 2019;**116**:4696-4705

[88] Welty S, Teng Y, Liang Z, Zhao W, Sanders LH, Greenamyre JT, et al. RAD52 is required for RNA-templated recombination repair in post-mitotic neurons. The Journal of Biological Chemistry. 2018;**293**:1353-1362

[89] Walker C, El-Khamisy SF. Perturbed autophagy and DNA repair converge to promote neurodegeneration in amyotrophic lateral sclerosis and dementia. Brain. 2018;**141**:1247-1262

[90] Pollari E, Goldsteins G, Bart G, Koistinaho J, Giniatullin R. The role of oxidative stress in degeneration of the neuromuscular junction in amyotrophic lateral sclerosis. Frontiers in Cellular Neuroscience. 2014;**8**:131

[91] Wang X, Michaelis EK. Selective neuronal vulnerability to oxidative stress in the brain. Frontiers in Aging Neuroscience. 2010;**2**:12

[92] Madabhushi R, Gao F, Pfenning AR, Pan L, Yamakawa S, Seo J, et al. Activity-induced DNA breaks govern the expression of neuronal early-response genes. Cell. 2015;**161**:1592-1605

[93] Kannan A, Bhatia K, Branzei D, Gangwani L. Combined deficiency of Senataxin and DNA-PKcs causes DNA damage accumulation and neurodegeneration in spinal muscular atrophy. Nucleic Acids Research. 2018;**46**:8326-8346

[94] Roda RH, Rinaldi C, Singh R, Schindler AB, Blackstone C. Ataxia with

oculomotor apraxia type 2 fibroblasts exhibit increased susceptibility to oxidative DNA damage. Journal of Clinical Neuroscience. 2014;**21**:1627-1631

[95] Storici F, Bebenek K, Kunkel TA, Gordenin DA, Resnick MA. RNA-templated DNA repair. Nature. 2007;**447**:338-341

[96] Keskin H, Shen Y, Huang F, Patel M, Yang T, Ashley K, et al. Transcript-RNA-templated DNA recombination and repair. Nature. 2014;**515**:436-439

[97] Wei W, Ba Z, Gao M, Wu Y, Ma Y, Amiard S, et al. A role for small RNAs in DNA double-strand break repair. Cell. 2012;**149**:101-112

[98] Wang Q, Goldstein M. Small RNAs recruit chromatin-modifying enzymes MMSET and Tip60 to reconfigure damaged DNA upon double-Strand break and facilitate repair. Cancer Research. 2016;**76**:1904-1915

[99] Gao M, Wei W, Li MM, Wu YS, Ba Z, Jin KX, et al. Ago2 facilitates Rad51 recruitment and DNA double-strand break repair by homologous recombination. Cell Research. 2014;**24**:532-541

[100] Ohle C, Tesorero R, Schermann G, Dobrev N, Sinning I, Fischer T. Transient RNA-DNA hybrids are required for efficient double-strand break repair. Cell. 2016;**167**:1001-1013

[101] Chakraborty A, Tapryal N, Venkova T, Horikoshi N, Pandita RK, Sarker AH, et al. Classical non-homologous end-joining pathway utilizes nascent RNA for error-free double-strand break repair of transcribed genes. Nature Communications. 2016;**7**:13049

[102] Francia S, Michelini F, Saxena A, Tang D, de Hoon M, Anelli V, et al. Site-specific DICER and DROSHA RNA products control the DNA-damage response. Nature. 2012;**488**:231-235

[103] Francia S, Cabrini M, Matti V, Oldani A, d'Adda di Fagagna F. DICER, DROSHA and DNA damage response RNAs are necessary for the secondary recruitment of DNA damage response factors. Journal of Cell Science. 2016;**129**:1468-1476

[104] Hamperl S, Cimprich KA. Conflict resolution in the genome: How transcription and replication make it work. Cell. 2016;**167**:1455-1467

[105] Alzu A, Bermejo R, Begnis M, Lucca C, Piccini D, Carotenuto W, et al. Senataxin associates with replication forks to protect fork integrity across RNA-polymerase-II-transcribed genes. Cell. 2012;**151**:835-846

[106] Eitan E, Hutchison ER, Mattson MP. Telomere shortening in neurological disorders: An abundance of unanswered questions. Trends in Neurosciences. 2014;**37**:256-263

[107] De Felice B, Annunziata A, Fiorentino G, Manfellotto F, D'Alessandro R, Marino R, et al. Telomerase expression in amyotrophic lateral sclerosis (ALS) patients. Journal of Human Genetics. 2014;**59**:555-561

[108] Cheng A, Shin-ya K, Wan R, Tang SC, Miura T, Tang H, et al. Telomere protection mechanisms change during neurogenesis and neuronal maturation: Newly generated neurons are hypersensitive to telomere and DNA damage. The Journal of Neuroscience. 2007;**27**:3722-3733

[109] Eitan E, Tichon A, Gazit A, Gitler D, Slavin S, Priel E. Novel telomerase-increasing compound in mouse brain delays the onset of amyotrophic lateral sclerosis. EMBO Molecular Medicine. 2012;**4**:313-329

[110] Zhu H, Fu W, Mattson MP. The catalytic subunit of telomerase protects neurons against amyloid beta-peptide-induced apoptosis. Journal of Neurochemistry. 2000;**75**:117-124

[111] De Amicis A, Piane M, Ferrari F, Fanciulli M, Delia D, Chessa L. Role of senataxin in DNA damage and telomeric stability. DNA Repair (Amst). 2011;**10**:199-209

[112] Foley NM, Hughes GM, Huang Z, Clarke M, Jebb D, Whelan CV, et al. Growing old, yet staying young: The role of telomeres in bats' exceptional longevity. Science Advances. 2018;**4**:eaao0926

[113] Grohmann K, Schuelke M, Diers A, Hoffmann K, Lucke B, Adams C, et al. Mutations in the gene encoding immunoglobulin mu-binding protein 2 cause spinal muscular atrophy with respiratory distress type 1. Nature Genetics. 2001;**29**:75-77

[114] Gama-Carvalho M, L Garcia-Vaquero M, R Pinto F, Besse F, Weis J, Voigt A, Schulz JB, De Las Rivas J. Linking amyotrophic lateral sclerosis and spinal muscular atrophy through RNA-transcriptome homeostasis: A genomics perspective. Journal of Neurochemistry. 2017;**141**:12-30

[115] Madabhushi R, Pan L, Tsai LH. DNA damage and its links to neurodegeneration. Neuron. 2014;**83**:266-282

[116] Konopka A, Atkin JD. The emerging role of DNA damage in the pathogenesis of the C9orf72 repeat expansion in amyotrophic lateral sclerosis. International Journal of Molecular Sciences. 2018;**19**:E3137

[117] Penndorf D, Witte OW, Kretz A. DNA plasticity and damage in amyotrophic lateral sclerosis. Neural Regeneration Research. 2018;**13**:173-180

[118] Wang H, Hegde ML. New mechanisms of DNA repair defects in fused in sarcoma-associated neurodegeneration: Stage set for DNA repair-based therapeutics? Journal of Experimental Neuroscience. 2019;**13**:1179069519856358

[119] Yeo AJ, Becherel OJ, Luff JE, Graham ME, Richard D, Lavin MF. Senataxin controls meiotic silencing through ATR activation and chromatin remodeling. Cell Discovery. 2015;**1**:15025

[120] Xue B, Dunbrack RL, Williams RW, Dunker AK, Uversky VN. PONDR-FIT: A meta-predictor of intrinsically disordered amino acids. Biochimica et Biophysica Acta. 2010;**1804**:996-1010

Chapter 4

Pathological Interaction between DNA Repair and Mitochondrial Dysfunction in ALS

Luis Bermúdez-Guzmán and Alejandro Leal

Abstract

Amyotrophic lateral sclerosis (ALS) is a neurodegenerative disease characterized by the degeneration of cortical and spinal cord motor neurons. Several mechanisms have been implicated in the pathogenesis of the disease, including mitochondrial dysfunction, oxidative stress, and genome instability. Recently, a combined role between impaired DNA repair and subsequent mitochondrial dysfunction has emerged as a novel pathological interaction in neurodegeneration. This is exemplified by mutations in the RNA-/DNA-binding proteins FUS and TDP-43 as well as superoxide dismutase 1 (SOD1) gene, all related to familial ALS. In this regard, evidence supports either downregulation or impaired recruitment of DNA repair enzymes in both nuclear and mitochondrial genomes. In addition, evidence also suggests a complex metabolic dysregulation as a critical component in the promotion of the disease. This chapter aims to integrate the molecular mechanisms of this pathological interplay and the possible role in cytosolic protein aggregation and cell death in motor neurons.

Keywords: DNA repair, neurodegeneration, mitochondria, motor neuron

1. Genome instability in the context of ALS pathogenesis

ALS has been traditionally classified as sporadic or familial (fALS). Specifically, four genes account for up to 70% of all cases of fALS: *C9orf72*, *TARDBP* (encoding TDP-43), *SOD1*, and *FUS*. Despite the Mendelian inheritance pattern, familial forms of ALS are usually characterized by incomplete penetrance, whereas genetic pleiotropy or oligogenic inheritance is suggested in individuals with sporadic disease [1]. Several hallmarks of neurodegeneration are shared in both familial and sporadic ALS, such as protein aggregation, defective autophagy, impaired DNA damage response (DDR), and mitochondrial dysfunction [1–3]. As ALS is a complex disease, it is plausible to think that regardless of the etiology, there is an interplay between these hallmarks in the pathogenesis and pathological progression.

Considering the late age of onset and the neurological tropism, which is the exclusive neurological affectation, it is possible to highlight some aspects of the nervous system that are useful to understand the molecular pathology of the disease. First, due to its high rate of oxygen consumption and metabolic activity, the nervous system is more susceptible to DNA damage [4]. Single-strand breaks (SSBs) are considered the most common damage to DNA in cells [5], mainly derived from reactive oxygen species [6]. Even physiological brain activity can also cause DNA double-strand breaks (DSBs) in neurons [7]. However, as neurons do not divide, homologous recombination (HR) is not available for DNA repair. In addition, to maintain normal functioning, neurons must ensure to keep mitochondrial homeostasis. Thus, there are different areas with high demands for ATP like synaptic terminals, active growth cones, or axonal branches that contain more mitochondria than other cellular domains [8, 9]. This dependency on mitochondrial homeostasis makes neurons more susceptible and more likely to be affected by mutations in genes regulating mitochondrial dynamics. For example, mutations in MFN2 and GDAP1 (which regulate mitochondrial fusion and fission, respectively) are related to Charcot-Marie-Tooth [10, 11], a peripheral neuropathy that resembles some of the clinical manifestations of ALS, especially in motor neurons. Thus, a disruption in normal nuclear and mitochondrial DNA (mtDNA) repair would affect motor neurons in a progressive way. Supporting this idea, several works have reported mtDNA mutations in presymptomatic animal models of ALS [12]. In fact, similar to CMT, mitochondrial axonal transportation has also been implicated in ALS. The SOD1-G93A mice showed alterations in the axonal traffic of mitochondria at a presymptomatic stage, specifically in motor neurons [13].

Interestingly, recent studies demonstrated that loss-of-function mutations in *KIF5A* are also a cause of ALS [14, 15]. *KIF5A* gene encodes for a specific motor protein implicated in the axonal transport of mitochondria. Although it was previously related with CMT and spastic paraplegia [16, 17], the new variants associated with ALS are primarily located at the C-terminal cargo-binding tail domain. Notably, patients harboring loss-of-function mutations displayed an extended survival relative to typical ALS cases.

A second aspect behind neurons' susceptibilities is their high rate of transcription. As they depend on the available DNA repair machinery, genomic stability is crucial for the maintenance of homeostasis. Transcription-driven DNA damage can arise from several sources, like the collapse of transcription machinery and subsequent DSBs, damage to genomic segments that have been opened up for transcription, and the formation of unnatural R-loop structures [18–21]. In the case of ALS cells, deficient DNA repair was reported more than three decades ago [22]. It seems that the DDR system in ALS loses adaptive capacity in dependency on the underlying genetic mutation [23]. The next chapter will address the role of the main genes involved in fALS in the generation of genomic instability as a hallmark of neurodegeneration.

2. Role of ALS-related genes in DDR

The hexanucleotide GGGGCC repeat expansion in *C9ORF72* is one of the most common genetic causes of both ALS and frontotemporal dementia (FTD). It was recently demonstrated that these expansions could cause defective DNA repair, manifested by higher levels of DSBs and impaired DDR [24]. Defective ATM-mediated DNA repair was found as a consequence of p62 accumulation, which impairs H2A ubiquitylation and perturbs ATM signaling. Another study reported that c-H2AX, p-ATM, 53BP1, and PARP1 were upregulated in C9orf72 patient spinal cords [25]. However, the mechanism behind the damage to the genome was not addressed. Authors suggest that R-loops, as well as the expression of dipeptide repeat proteins, are more likely to be the cause. Consistent with this notion, elevated levels of DNA damage markers γH2AX, ATR, GADD45, and p53 were present in motor neurons differentiated from iPSC lines from C9orf72-mutant ALS patients in response to oxidative stress [26].

In a model of C9orf72-induced ALS, the overexpression of SETX or depletion of p62 was capable of reducing γH2AX foci in MRC5 cells. In fact, the combined overexpression of SETX and depletion of p62 further reduced DSB levels compared to levels observed by SETX overexpression or p62 depletion alone [24]. Interestingly, mutations in SETX cause both ataxia with oculomotor apraxia type 2 (AOA2) (autosomal recessive) and amyotrophic lateral sclerosis 4 (ALS4) (autosomal dominant). The N-terminal protein interaction and C-terminal RNA/DNA helicase domains are conserved in the *Saccharomyces cerevisiae* SETX homolog Sen1p. In a mutant model of Sen1p in *S. cerevisiae,* alterations in redox state, unfolded protein response, TOR, and severe loss of mitochondrial DNA were demonstrated [27].

Other ALS-related genes can cause DNA damage. The cytoplasmic inclusions of TDP-43 and FUS seen in ALS can be derived from a toxic gain of function, which, in turn, triggers motor neuron cell death [18]. As the majority of ALS-causing mutations are located within the C-terminus of FUS, it has been suggested that these mutations impair the DNA pairing function of FUS, compromising genome stability [28]. Moreover, depletion of either FUS or TDP-43 in cells treated with α-amanitin (an RNA Pol II inhibitor) led to higher DNA strand breaks [18]. It also was demonstrated that after UV damage-induced transcription arrest, FUS localizes at genomic sites where active transcription has been arrested by DNA damage, and it does so together with BRCA1 [18]. TDP-43 is also able to localize at sites of transcription-associated DNA damage, given its colocalization with γH2AX and phosphorylated RPA. Interestingly, TDP-43 also colocalized with γH2AX and phosphorylated RPA in undamaged cells, consistent with its role in preventing or repairing spontaneously arising DNA damage [18].

FUS and TDP-43 are also required to maintain R-loop homeostasis since their depletion leads to R-loop-mediated genomic instability [29]. It is speculated that RNA processing factors prevent R-loop by binding to the nascent RNA transcript and blocking R-loop formation. In this regard, it has been shown that FUS and TDP-43 colocalize with active RNA polymerase II at sites of DNA damage along with BRCA1, either to prevent or repair R-loop-associated DNA damage, normally considered an indicator of defective transcription and/or RNA processing [18].

3. Mitochondrial dysfunction in ALS

The space-time location of mitochondria is vital for the metabolic requirements of the nervous system, especially in the case of motor neurons. As neurons cannot rely on glycolysis, mitochondria are crucial to meet the high energy demands mainly by oxidative phosphorylation (OXPHOS). Several aspects of mitochondrial dynamics have been involved in the pathogenesis of ALS. For example, ATP generation was markedly decreased in neuronal cells of mutant SOD1-G93A mice [30, 31]. Moreover, cytosolic ATP levels were significantly reduced in neuroblastoma cells expressing mutant SOD1-G37R and in rotenone-treated SOD1-G93A neuronal cells [32]. Impairment of intracellular Ca^{2+} homeostasis is also considered as a hallmark of mitochondrial dysfunction in neurodegeneration. In this regard, an imbalance in Ca^{2+} dynamics has been reported in cells expressing both mutant SOD1-G93A and SOD1-G37R [33, 34] and in motor neurons from mutant SOD1-G93A transgenic mice [35].

Mitochondrial fusion and fission are also key processes to preserve organelle functioning and cellular homeostasis. Dynamin-related protein 1 (Drp1) influences cell survival and apoptosis by mediating the mitochondrial fission process in mammals [36]. An excessive mitochondrial fragmentation and dysfunction were reported in patient-derived fibroblasts and cultured motor neurons of several familial forms of ALS expressing SOD1 mutant [37]. In the same article, authors demonstrated that inhibition of Drp1/Fis1 interaction led to a significant reduction in ROS levels and improved mitochondrial function and structure. Mutations in SOD1, TARDBP, or FUS are related to protein aggregation. In this regard, aggregated proteins can also contribute to mitochondrial dysfunction. Moreover, ATP decrease and ROS increase are the main features of mitochondrial damage. While ROS can increase Drp1 leading to sustained mitochondrial fission and fragmentation, a decrease in ATP levels can impair autophagy and proteasomal degradation. This can worsen protein aggregates and trigger ER stress [37, 38].

More than two decades ago, Kong and Xu reported that in mice expressing SOD1-G93A, the onset of the disease involved a decline of muscle strength and a transient explosive increase in vacuoles derived from degenerating mitochondria. Interestingly, this damage did not involve motor neuron death at the time of onset. Based on their results, the authors suggested that SOD1-mutant toxicity was mediated by damage to mitochondria in motor neurons [39]. The early findings of mitochondrial dysfunction were also confirmed by Magrané and colleagues, who studied the mitochondrial transport within the sciatic nerve in SOD1-G93A and TDP-43-A315T mice. Defects of retrograde mitochondrial transport were detected at 45 days of age in both mice, before the onset of symptoms [40]. In the SOD1-G93A mice, mitochondrial morphological abnormalities were apparent at day 15 of age, thus preceding transport abnormalities. Conversely, in TDP-43-A315T mice, morphological abnormalities appeared after the onset of transport defects. Interestingly, the authors reported neither morphological nor mitochondrial distribution changes in sensory neurons [40].

Another study evaluated the role of SOD1 mutations in mitochondrial homeostasis, in spinal cord sections from early symptomatic 10-month mice. Authors showed that mutant SOD1 binding to mitochondria disrupts normal distribution and morphology as an early pathogenic feature. In their work, mitochondria from SOD G85R/G37R mice became progressively smaller and rounder and are unevenly distributed along axons [41]. As in SOD1 mutant experiments, oxidative stress and DNA damage were increased in iPSC-derived C9ORF72 motor neurons in an age-dependent manner [26]. Poly (GR) preferentially binds to mitochondrial ribosomal proteins and compromised mitochondrial function, which could lead to increased oxidative stress. Reducing oxidative stress partially rescued DNA damage in C9ORF72 motor neurons cells [26].

The role of mutant FUS and TDP-43 has also been evaluated in mitochondrial dysfunction. In cultured neurons expressing FUS-R495X, it was revealed that mutant FUS controlled the translation of genes that were associated with mitochondria function, which resulted in a significant reduction of mitochondrial size [42]. Specifically, protein levels of KIF5B, DNM1L, and CSDE1 were significantly reduced in R495X-expressing neurons. FUS is also able to translocate and accumulate inside mitochondria. Following this approach, it was revealed that FUS could interact with mitochondrial chaperonin HSP60 and this interaction mediates FUS localization to the organelle, leading to damage [43]. This damage derives from reduced mitochondrial membrane potential and increased production of ROS. Authors also reported elevated HSP60 expression in two of three cases of FTLD-FUS patients' brain samples. Curiously, mutations in the *HSPD1* gene which encodes for HSP60 protein have also been found in patients with spastic paraplegia type 13 [44]. Another work revealed that mitochondrial impairment is a critical early event in FUS proteinopathy. When mutant FUS-P525L accumulated inside mitochondria, it interacted with the mitochondrial ATP synthase catalytic subunit ATP5B and reduced mitochondrial ATP synthesis. Importantly, FUS accumulation also induced the mitochondrial unfolded protein response (UPTmt), making the damage even worse [45].

Similarly, mutant TDP-43 accumulates in the mitochondria of neurons in subjects with ALS or frontotemporal dementia (FTD). Wild-type and mutant TDP-43 preferentially bind to mitochondria-transcribed mRNAs encoding respiratory complex I subunits ND3/ND6, causing complex I disassembly [46]. The suppression of TDP-43 mitochondrial localization abolished mitochondrial dysfunction and neuronal loss and improved the phenotypes of transgenic mutant TDP-43 mice. Mutant FUS can also alter mitochondrial-endoplasmic reticulum (ER) communication. Stoica and colleagues showed that FUS disrupts the VAPB-PTPIP51 complex, impairing ER-mitochondria association. As a consequence, there was a perturbation of Ca^{2+} uptake by mitochondria and impaired ATP production [47]. Remarkably, inhibition of glycogen synthase kinase-3b (GSK-3b) corrected FUS-induced defects in ER-mitochondria associations and mitochondrial Ca^{2+} levels.

Mitochondrial DNA damage is also important in the context of neurodegenerative diseases [48, 49]. Maintaining mitochondrial DNA stability is critical for cellular function, especially in the context of the nervous system. Several pathways have been implicated in mtDNA repair, but base excision repair (BER) is the predominant one [50]. Oxoguanine glycosylase 1 (OGG1) is an enzyme that plays a major role in the mitochondrial BER pathway, removing 8-hydroxy-2-deoxyguanosine (8-OHdG). In the spinal cord of SOD1 mutant transgenic mice, the presence of 8-OHdG was progressively accumulated in the ventral horn neurons from early and presymptomatic stage (25 weeks) [51]. This was a suggestion that an oxidative damage to mitochondrial DNA was affecting spinal motor neurons at a very early stage of the disease. Early and selective impairment of DNA repair enzymes in mitochondria was also reported in presymptomatic transgenic mice carrying a mutant SOD1 gene [51]. Notably, the selective expression of these enzymes in spinal neurons is closely related to the selective involvement of motor neurons in ALS.

In the ALS but not control brains, levels of a common mitochondrial DNA deletion mutation (mt DNA4977) were an average of more than 30-fold in Brodmann area 4 [52]. In addition, the oxidative damage derived from 8-oxoG was accumulated in the mitochondria of motor neurons in ALS, and according to previous findings, OGG1 did not repair the damage efficiently, driving the loss of motor neurons in ALS [53]. Likewise, motor neurons in G93A-mSOD1 transgenic mice undergo slow degeneration characterized by mitochondrial swelling and formation of DNA single-strand breaks prior to double-strand breaks occurring in both nuclear and mitochondrial DNA [54]. These cells accumulated mitochondria from the axon terminals and generated higher levels of ROS/RNS. Despite experimental evidence demonstrating mtDNA damage, more research is required to elucidate the mechanisms that lead to mitochondrial damage in ALS. The mechanisms that can link the DNA repair deficiency induced by errors in ALS-associated proteins and the subsequent mitochondrial dysfunction in terms of genetic integrity are not yet understood. We believe that this is an issue that should be taken into account for future studies.

4. Nuclear-mitochondrial interplay and genomic integrity in ALS

4.1 The role of SIRT1-PARP1 axis

Poly (ADP-ribose) polymerase 1 (PARP1) is a NAD+-dependent protein. It is able to posttranslationally modify itself and other proteins involved in multiple DDR. PARP1 is also crucial for the stabilization of DNA replication forks and chromatin remodeling [55]. Deletion of *Parp1* gene in *Xrcc1* knockout mice is able to prevent neurodegeneration, indicating that the overactivation of PARP1 is a neurotoxic consequence of defective DNA repair [56]. Recently, it was demonstrated that FUS can bind directly to PAR, the polymer made by PARP1 [57]. Authors revealed that FUS is recruited to chromosomal sites of oxidative DNA damage and that this recruitment is reduced by the FUS-R521G mutation. Additionally, when cells lack PARP1, FUS failed to accumulate at sites of UVA laser-induced damage. Moreover, under oxidative stress, PARP1 activity increases, leading to an accumulation of ADP-ribose polymers and NAD+ depletion. This condition induces a metabolic and energetic crisis driving cell death [58]. As PARP1 hyperactivation and toxicity have been implicated in diseases like Alzheimer's, Parkinson's, and Huntington's, a predominant role in ALS is also plausible [59].

Sirtuins are also NAD-dependent proteins. SIRT1 is known as a nuclear and cytoplasmic deacetylase, which is predominantly expressed in neurons in the context of the nervous system [60]. Notably, PARP1 consumes NAD+, reducing SIRT1 activity by increasing PARylation of DNA and proteins involved in DDR. Thus, SIRT1 activity appears to be impeded by PARP1 hyperactivation [61]. Interestingly, NAD+ replenishment shows a reactivation of SIRT1 and prevented neurodegeneration [62]. Thus, compromised DNA repair leads to PARP1 hyperactivation, resulting in the depletion of NAD+ levels, inhibiting SIRTs (**Figure 1**). Notably, the Km of SIRT1 for NAD+ is higher than that of PARP1, so when NAD+ levels become so low following cell stress or senescence, SIRT1 no longer has the chance to regulate the activity of PARP1 [61]. Cantó and colleagues demonstrated that deletion of *Parp1* gene increased NAD+ levels and SIRT1 activity in brown adipose tissue and muscle. *Parp1 −/−* mice presented a higher mitochondrial content, resulting in increased energy expenditure and protection against metabolic disease. As previously reported, authors showed that pharmacologic inhibition of PARP in vitro and in vivo increased NAD+, leading to SIRT1 expression and enhanced oxidative metabolism [63].

SIRT1 is vital in the maintenance of metabolic homeostasis [64]. SIRT1 can activate the peroxisome proliferator-activated receptor γ (PPARγ) coactivator-1α (PGC-1α) through deacetylation [65]. PGC-1a can regulate genes of the ROS defense system. It has been shown that PGC-1a can protect WT neural cells from oxidative stress by increasing the expression of ROS-detoxifying genes including SOD1/SOD2 and UCP2 [66]. SIRT1 may also deacetylate PGC-1α to induce mitochondrial biogenesis by increasing mitochondrial gene expression via nuclear respiratory factor 1 (NRF-1) and nuclear-encoded mitochondrial transcription factor A (TFAM) [67]. Interestingly, it was revealed that PGC-1 and SIRT1 are also present inside the mitochondria and are in close proximity to mtDNA [68]. In addition, an unexpected role for serotonin (5-HT) was also recently demonstrated. Fanibunda and colleagues showed that in rodent cortical neurons, serotonin is a regulator of mitochondrial biogenesis, via 5-HT2A receptor-mediated recruitment of the SIRT1-PGC-1α axis [69].

SIRT1 can form a protein complex with the Forkhead transcription factor FOXO3 and promote its deacetylation. SIRT1 induces several effects mediated by FOXO3 like cell cycle arrest and transcription of DNA repair target genes [70]. Cantó and colleagues demonstrated that AMPK enhances SIRT1 activity by increasing cellular NAD+ levels [71]. This resulted in the deacetylation and modulation of the activity of downstream SIRT1 targets including PGC-11α and FOXO1/FOXO3a transcription factors. Thus, SIRT1 could promote both mitochondrial biogenesis in conditions of energy deficiency in disease or induce the clearance of damaged mitochondria [72].

In XPA-deficient cells, a model of xeroderma pigmentosum, the DNA repair deficiency leads to PARP1 activation, and the attenuated NAD+/SIRT1/PGC-1α axis resulted in defective mitophagy. The condition could be rescued either by

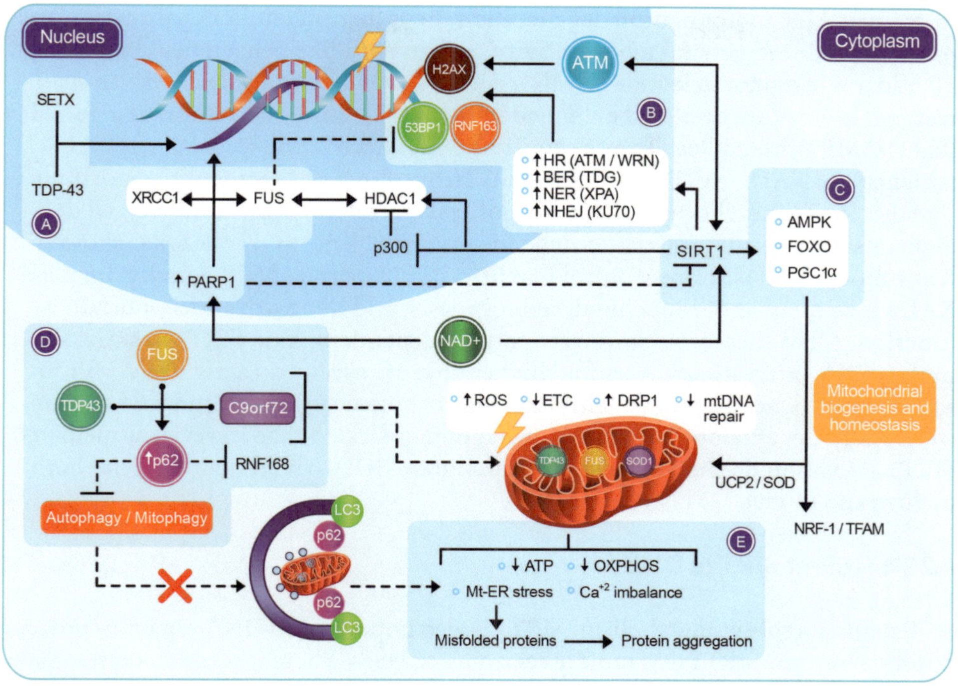

Figure 1.
Nuclear-mitochondrial interplay in the context of ALS. (A) Activation of PARP1 upon DNA damage facilitates DNA repair but inhibits SIRT1 due to NAD+ depletion. FUS binds directly to PAR, the polymer made by PARP1 in chromosomal sites of oxidative DNA damage. Both TDP-43 and FUS localize at genomic sites where active transcription has been arrested by DNA damage and also maintain R-loop homeostasis. SETX is also necessary for R-loop repair. In addition, FUS interacts with HDAC1 and enhances its activity in both physiological conditions and DNA damage. (B) SIRT1 positively regulates DDR. SIRT is able to deacetylase HDAC1, ATM, WRN, TDG, XPA, and KU70. (C) SIRT1 also regulates mitochondrial homeostasis through AMPK, FOXOs, and PGC1α. These enzymes regulate mitochondrial biogenesis and oxidative stress, transcribing proteins such as UCP2 and SODs. (D) Accumulation of misfolded proteins leads to the aberrant p62 expression, disrupting normal mitophagy. Likewise, defective ATM-mediated DNA repair is a consequence of p62 accumulation and RNF168 inhibition. C9orf72 can also cause defective DNA repair and p62 accumulation with the subsequent impaired mitophagy. (E) ALS-related mitochondrial dysfunction leads to mitochondrial fragmentation through DRP1 overexpression, decreased ATP production, higher ROS levels, mtDNA damage, decrease in OXPHOS, and Ca^{+2} imbalance. FUS can accumulate inside the mitochondria, leading to impaired ATP production and increased ROS levels. C9ORF72 can also generate oxidative stress and mtDNA damage in motor neurons. TDP-43 preferentially bind to mitochondria-transcribed mRNAs, causing complex I disassembly. SOD1 mutations can decrease cytosolic ATP levels, impair intracellular Ca^{2+} homeostasis, generate excessive mitochondrial fragmentation, and deregulate DDR. The final effect of this cascade is derived from mitochondria-ER stress, consequent misfolded proteins, and further protein aggregation. Dotted lines illustrate pathological interactions.

PARP1 inhibition or by supplementation with NAD+ [73]. In a different work, Scheibye-Knudsen and colleagues showed that hyperactivation of PARP1 drives SIRT1 depression in Cockayne syndrome (CS). Similar to previous findings, NAD+ replenishment rescued the phenotype in CS, but in this case, they also demonstrated that diet can also increase SIRT1 activity [62]. Following the same line, it was revealed that NAD+ levels are reduced in aged mice and *Caenorhabditis elegans* [74]. Genetic or pharmacological restoration of NAD+ prevented age-associated metabolic decline and promoted longevity in worms. These effects were associated with deacetylase sir-2.1 levels, the homolog of SIRT1. Indeed, hyperacetylation of the SIRT1 substrate PGC-1α resulted from low levels of NAD+ in aged mice [74]. Supporting this approach, it was demonstrated that the intracellular nicotinamide phosphoribosyltransferase (iNAMPT) is essential to projection neuron function and viability. The iNAMPT is the rate-limiting enzyme of the mammalian NAD+ biosynthesis. When eliminating *Nampt* in adult mice, the resulting phenotype resembled ALS: motor neuron degeneration, hypothermia, motor dysfunction and paralysis, reduced general motor activity, and anxiety-like behaviors. Remarkably, nicotinamide mononucleotide (NMN), a NAD+ precursor, improved health span, restored motor function, and extended lifespan [75]. Since the authors also found that iNAMPT protein levels were significantly reduced in the spinal cord of ALS patients, the NAD+/SIRT1 axis represents an outstanding therapeutic opportunity.

For a long time, the beneficial effect of resveratrol has been controversial due to inconsistent results and tissue-dependent effects. Price and colleagues showed that a moderate dose of resveratrol is able to stimulate the AMPK activity, increase NAD+ levels, enhance mitochondrial biogenesis, and improve mitochondrial function. All of these functions were entirely dependent upon SIRT1 in skeletal muscle [76]. Interestingly, a tenfold higher dose of resveratrol activated AMPK in a SIRT1-independent manner, although improvements in mitochondrial function were SIRT1 dependent [76]. Finally, it was demonstrated that resveratrol-mediated SIRT1 activation protects against p25 and mutant SOD1-G93A neurotoxicity both in vitro and in vivo [77].

4.2 The role of SIRT in DDR

Beyond its role in metabolism, SIRT1 is also important in DNA repair. In post-mitotic neurons, SIRT1 was rapidly recruited to DSBs where it showed a synergistic relationship with ATM, stimulating its autophosphorylation and stabilizing ATM at DSBs' sites [78]. Additionally, authors reported that after DSBs' induction, SIRT1 also bound HDAC1, a neuroprotective histone deacetylase, stimulating its enzymatic activity. This activity is necessary for the nonhomologous end joining (NHEJ) pathway [78]. Likewise, upon exposure to radiation, SIRT1 can enhance DNA repair capacity and deacetylation of repair protein Ku70, involved in NHEJ as well [79].

SIRT1 also interacts with WRN both in vitro and in vivo, and this interaction is enhanced after DNA damage [80]. WRN is a member of the RecQ DNA helicase family with functions in maintaining genome stability. Moreover, the MRE11-RAD50-NBS1 (MRN) is a conserved nuclease complex that exhibits properties of a DNA damage sensor in the context of DSBs. SIRT1 can associate with the MRN complex and maintains NBS1 in a hypoacetylated state following ionizing radiation [81]. SIRT1 is also important for the base excision repair (BER) pathway. It was shown that SIRT1 deacetylates APE1 in vitro and in vivo following genotoxic insults [82]. Knockdown of SIRT1 increases cellular abasic DNA content, sensitizing cells to death induced by genotoxic stress. Interestingly, the activation of SIRT1 with resveratrol promoted binding of APE1 to XRCC1 [82]. Thymine DNA glycosylase (TDG) is an essential multifunctional enzyme also involved in BER. SIRT1 was shown to interact with TDG and enhance its glycosylase activity due to deacetylation [83]. Nucleotide excision repair (NER) is another important pathway in DNA repair. NER removes DNA damage induced by ultraviolet light (UV). Xeroderma pigmentosum group A (XPA) is a critical protein for this process. SIRT1 interacts with XPA, and the interaction is enhanced after UV irradiation [84]. In fact, down-regulation of SIRT1 sensitized cells to UV irradiation.

4.3 The role of FUS in DDR

FUS is important for both NHEJ- and HR-mediated DSB repair in neurons. As SIRT1, FUS interacts with HDAC1 and enhances its activity in both physiological conditions and DNA damage in cortical neurons [85]. The same was demonstrated in human-induced pluripotent stem cells (hiPSCs) and hiPSC-derived motor neurons. The degree of FUS mislocalization correlated well with the clinical severity of the underlying ALS, with a higher accumulation of DNA damage in postmitotic mutated FUS motor neurons than in dividing hiPSCs [86]. Although FUS has been associated with multiple DNA repair pathways including DSB repair, quantification of the level of DNA SSBs vs. DSBs in FUS knockdown (KD) and knockout (KO) cells by comet analysis revealed that most unrepaired DNA strand breaks that accumulated after the loss of FUS were SSBs [87].

FUS protects the genome by facilitating PARP1-dependent recruitment of XRCC1/DNA ligase IIIα (LigIII) to oxidized genome sites and activating LigIII via direct interaction [88]. Cells presenting mutant FUS showed a significantly reduced association between this DNA repair protein complex, SSBs' accumulation, and ROS levels in motor neurons. LigIII was demonstrated to be an essential enzyme for mtDNA integrity but dispensable for nuclear DNA repair [89]. LigI was critical for nuclear DNA repair in a cooperative manner with LigIII, but inactivation of LigIII resulted in mtDNA loss, mitochondrial dysfunction, and incapacitating ataxia in the mouse nervous system. However, as neurons do not divide, it is possible that LigIII is equally important for nuclear DNA repair. Following the idea that mtDNA integrity is vital in postmitotic tissues, the authors also found that inactivation of LigIII in cardiac muscle resulted in mitochondrial dysfunction and defective heart-pump function leading to heart failure [89]. More research is needed to elucidate the interaction of ALS-associated proteins with both nuclear and mitochondrial DNA repair enzymes (**Figure 1**).

4.4 Cross talk between auto-/mitophagy and DNA repair in ALS

Autophagy is a crucial process to eliminate misfolded proteins and organelles. Mitophagy is a special subroutine of autophagy, involved in the maintenance of mitochondrial homeostasis. An important protein regulating this process is p62. The molecular mechanism of p62-mediated mitochondrial defective clearance was demonstrated by Geisler and colleagues [90]. Knockdown of p62 significantly diminished mitochondria recognition by the autophagy machinery and its subsequent elimination [91]. Notably, accumulation of misfolded proteins leads to the aberrant p62 expression, which influences the balance of mitophagy, worsens mitochondrial dysfunction, and induces more protein aggregates [92]. This can explain the vulnerability of non-cycling cells to proteinopathies in the context of mitochondrial dysfunction [93–96].

Autophagy is also important to maintain functional DNA repair by preventing p62 accumulation. In the context of ALS, where p62 accumulates, RNF168-mediated H2A ubiquitylation (U) is perturbed, leading to impaired DSBs' repair and genomic instability [29]. Wang and colleagues reported that p62/SQSTM1, which accumulates in autophagy-defective cells, directly binds to and inhibits nuclear RNF168, which is crucial for histone H2A ubiquitination and DNA damage responses. As a result, DNA repair proteins such as BRCA1, RAP80, and Rad51 cannot be recruited to the sites of DNA double-strand breaks (DSBs), which impairs DSBs' repair [97]. The interaction between mitochondrial dysfunction, defective mitophagy, and protein aggregation should be the subject of further investigation. This could generate new therapeutic avenues in the context of neurodegenerative diseases that occur with proteinopathies.

5. Therapeutic challenges and opportunities

Despite the clear role of mitochondria in neurodegeneration, the application of translational medicine in this field remains to be addressed. The lack of new therapeutic options and the limitations of current genetic editing techniques make it difficult to have a clear path for future research. Due to the failure in targeting specific aspects of mitochondria, mitochondrial transplantation presents a new paradigm of therapeutic intervention that may benefit neuronal survival and regeneration in ALS and similar diseases. The clinical application of mitochondrial transplantation was extensively reviewed by Chang and colleagues already [98].

The importance of this approach has been demonstrated in different lines of research. For example, it was shown that astrocytes in mice release functional mitochondria that enter neurons and amplify cell survival signals after stroke [99]. Cardiomyocytes share several similitudes with neurons, including the postmitotic state, the high transcription rate, the similar metabolic profile, and the underlying dependence on mitochondrial homeostasis. Following myocardial ischemia and reperfusion (IR), several alterations have been demonstrated in mitochondrial structure and function. Mitochondrial transplantation has been proposed as a strong opportunity for the treatment of IR [100]. Masuzawa and colleagues showed in a model of ischemia-reperfusion injury that transplantation of autologously derived mitochondria immediately prior to reperfusion ameliorated the damage. By using New Zealand white rabbits, they demonstrated a complete recovery and showed that the transplanted mitochondria enhanced oxygen consumption, high-energy phosphate synthesis, and enhanced post-infarct cardiac function [101].

In a model of Parkinson's disease induced by the respiratory chain inhibitor MPTP, Shi and colleagues demonstrated in mice that intravenous injection of mitochondria prevented the progression of the disease. Specifically, the authors reported increased activity of the electron transport chain, decreased ROS levels, and prevention of cell apoptosis and necrosis [102]. Other approaches have been addressed following this so-called mitochondrial medicine approach in ALS, such as ketogenic diet, antioxidants, and metabolic targeting drugs [103]. Based on the evidence provided until this point, mitochondrial transplantation should be validated as a therapeutic option in ALS. The safety and efficacy, delivery strategies, the periodicity of the transplant, and the capture by the cells of interest should be rigorously analyzed experimentally. Thus, if its effectiveness is proven in animal models, hopefully, clinical trials can be performed soon.

6. Conclusions

The DNA repair deficiency is a hallmark that combines at the pathological level with mitochondrial dysfunction, which highlights the special dependence of neurons on genomic integrity and metabolic stability. This highlights what we called the pathological tropism of the nervous system. At this point, it is clear that whatever the etiology behind ALS and motor neuron degeneration, mitochondrial dysfunction is present in all fALS and sporadic ALS patients. The fact that mitochondrial damage appears in the presymptomatic stage of the disease raises an opportunity for targeting mitochondria and hopefully makes disease progression slower or even stops it. Mitochondrial transplantation represents a promising avenue for the following years, as well as NAD+ repletion therapy and mitophagy-inducing agents.

Acknowledgements

We acknowledge the support from the University of Costa Rica (project 111-B2–372). We also thank Gabriel Jiménez Huezo for the graphic design of the picture in this chapter.

Conflict of interest

The authors declare no conflict of interests.

Nomenclature

ALS	amyotrophic lateral sclerosis
fALS	familial amyotrophic lateral sclerosis
DDR	DNA damage response
DSBs	double-strand breaks
NAD+	nicotinamide adenine dinucleotide
SETX	senataxin
ROS	reactive oxygen species
RNS	reactive nitrogen species
NHEJ	nonhomologous end joining
BER	base excision repair
SIRT	Sirtuin 1
FUS	fused in sarcoma
HDAC1	histone deacetylase 1
HiPSCs	human-induced pluripotent stem cells
PARP1	poly (ADP-ribose) polymerase 1
XRCC1	X-ray repair cross-complementing 1
TDP-43	TAR DNA-binding protein 43
SOD1	superoxide dismutase 1
C9orf72	chromosome 9 open reading frame 72
SSBs	single-strand breaks
HR	homologous recombination
MFN2	mitofusin 2
GDAP1	ganglioside-induced differentiation-associated protein 1
mtDNA	mitochondrial DNA
KIF5A	kinesin heavy chain isoform 5A
ATM	ataxia telangiectasia mutated
53BP1	p53-binding protein 1
UPRmt	mitochondrial unfolded protein response
FTD	frontotemporal dementia
ER	endoplasmic reticulum
GSK-3b	glycogen synthase kinase-3b
PGC-1α	peroxisome proliferator-activated receptor gamma coactivator-1 alpha
iNAMPT	intracellular nicotinamide phosphoribosyltransferase
NMN	nicotinamide mononucleotide
RNF168	RING-type E3 ubiquitin transferase
BRCA1	breast cancer 1
MPTP	1-methyl-4-phenyl-1,2,3,6-tetrahydropyridine
AMPK	MP-activated protein kinase
FOXOs	forkhead box O proteins

Author details

Luis Bermúdez-Guzmán[1] and Alejandro Leal[1,2*]

1 Section of Genetics and Biotechnology, School of Biology, Universidad de Costa Rica, San José, Costa Rica

2 Neuroscience Research Center, Universidad de Costa Rica, San José, Costa Rica

*Address all correspondence to: alejandro.leal@ucr.ac.cr

References

[1] Hardiman O, Al-Chalabi A, Chio A, Corr EM, Logroscino G, Robberecht W, et al. Amyotrophic lateral sclerosis. Nature Reviews. Disease Primers. 2017;**3**:17071. DOI: 10.1038/nrdp.2017.71

[2] Morgan S, Orrell RW. Pathogenesis of amyotrophic lateral sclerosis. British Medical Bulletin. 2016;**119**:87-98. DOI: 10.1093/bmb/ldw026

[3] Jiang Z, Wang W, Perry G, Zhu X, Wang X. Mitochondrial dynamic abnormalities in amyotrophic lateral sclerosis. Translational Neurodegeneration. 2015;**4**:14. DOI: 10.1186/s40035-015-0037-x

[4] Barzilai A. The contribution of the DNA damage response to neuronal viability. Antioxidants and Redox Signaling. 2007;**9**:211-218. DOI: 10.1089/ars.2007.9.211

[5] Caldecott KW. Single-strand break repair and genetic disease. Nature Reviews. Genetics. 2008;**9**:619-631. DOI: 10.1038/nrg2380

[6] Tann AW, Boldogh I, Meiss G, Qian W, Van Houten B, Mitra S, et al. Apoptosis induced by persistent single-strand breaks in mitochondrial genome: Critical role of EXOG (5′-EXO/endonuclease) in their repair. The Journal of Biological Chemistry. 2011;**286**:31975-31983. DOI: 10.1074/jbc.M110.215715

[7] Suberbielle E, Sanchez PE, Kravitz AV, Wang X, Ho K, Eilertson K, et al. Physiologic brain activity causes DNA double-strand breaks in neurons, with exacerbation by amyloid-β. Nature Neuroscience. 2013;**16**:613-621. DOI: 10.1038/nn.3356

[8] Sajic M, Mastrolia V, Lee CY, Trigo D, Sadeghian M, Mosley AJ, et al. Impulse conduction increases mitochondrial transport in adult mammalian peripheral nerves in vivo. PLoS Biology. 2013;**11**:e1001754. DOI: 10.1371/journal.pbio.1001754

[9] Misgeld T, Schwarz TL. Mitostasis in neurons: Maintaining mitochondria in an extended cellular architecture. Neuron. 2017;**96**:651-666. DOI: 10.1016/j.neuron.2017.09.055

[10] Niemann A, Wagner KM, Ruegg M, Suter U. GDAP1 mutations differ in their effects on mitochondrial dynamics and apoptosis depending on the mode of inheritance. Neurobiology of Disease. 2009;**36**:509-520. DOI: 10.1016/j.nbd.2009.09.011

[11] Zhou Y, Carmona S, Muhammad AKMG, Bell S, Landeros J, Vazquez M, et al. Restoring mitofusin balance prevents axonal degeneration in a Charcot-Marie-Tooth type 2A model. Journal of Clinical Investigation. 2019;**129**:1756-1771. DOI: 10.1172/JCI124194

[12] Cha M-Y, Kim DK, Mook-Jung I. The role of mitochondrial DNA mutation on neurodegenerative diseases. Experimental and Molecular Medicine. 2015;**47**:e150-e150. DOI: 10.1038/emm.2014.122

[13] Bilsland LG, Sahai E, Kelly G, Golding M, Greensmith L, Schiavo G. Deficits in axonal transport precede ALS symptoms in vivo. Proceedings of the National Academy of Sciences. 2010;**107**:20523-20528. DOI: 10.1073/pnas.1006869107

[14] Nicolas A, Kenna KP, Renton AE, Ticozzi N, Faghri F, Chia R, et al. Genome-wide analyses identify KIF5A as a novel ALS gene. Neuron. 2018;**97**:1268-1283.e6. DOI: 10.1016/j.neuron.2018.02.027

[15] Brenner D, Yilmaz R, Müller K, Grehl T, Petri S, Meyer T, et al.

Hot-spot KIF5A mutations cause familial ALS. Brain. 2018;**141**:688-697. DOI: 10.1093/brain/awx370

[16] Goizet C, Boukhris A, Mundwiller E, Tallaksen C, Forlani S, Toutain A, et al. Complicated forms of autosomal dominant hereditary spastic paraplegia are frequent in SPG10. Human Mutation. 2009;**30**:E376-E385. DOI: 10.1002/humu.20920

[17] Crimella C, Baschirotto C, Arnoldi A, Tonelli A, Tenderini E, Airoldi G, et al. Mutations in the motor and stalk domains of KIF5A in spastic paraplegia type 10 and in axonal Charcot-Marie-Tooth type 2. Clinical Genetics. 2012;**82**:157-164. DOI: 10.1111/j.1399-0004.2011.01717.x

[18] Hill SJ, Mordes DA, Cameron LA, Neuberg DS, Landini S, Eggan K, et al. Two familial ALS proteins function in prevention/repair of transcription-associated DNA damage. Proceedings of the National Academy of Sciences of the United States of America. 2016;**113**:E7701-E7709. DOI: 10.1073/pnas.1611673113

[19] Aguilera A, García-Muse T. R loops: From transcription byproducts to threats to genome stability. Molecular Cell. 2012;**46**:115-124. DOI: 10.1016/j.molcel.2012.04.009

[20] Skourti-Stathaki K, Proudfoot NJ. A double-edged sword: R loops as threats to genome integrity and powerful regulators of gene expression. Genes and Development. 2014;**28**:1384-1396. DOI: 10.1101/gad.242990.114

[21] Paulsen RD, Soni DV, Wollman R, Hahn AT, Yee M-C, Guan A, et al. A genome-wide siRNA screen reveals diverse cellular processes and pathways that mediate genome stability. Molecular Cell. 2009;**35**:228-239. DOI: 10.1016/j.molcel.2009.06.021

[22] Tandan R, Robison SH, Munzer JS, Bradley WG. Deficient DNA repair in amyotrophic lateral sclerosis cells. Journal of the Neurological Sciences. 1987;**79**:189-203. DOI: 10.1016/0022-510X(87)90272-3

[23] Coppedè F. An overview of DNA repair in amyotrophic lateral sclerosis. The Scientific World Journal. 2011;**11**:1679-1691. DOI: 10.1100/2011/853474

[24] Walker C, Herranz-Martin S, Karyka E, Liao C, Lewis K, Elsayed W, et al. C9orf72 expansion disrupts ATM-mediated chromosomal break repair. Nature Neuroscience. 2017;**20**:1225-1235. DOI: 10.1038/nn.4604

[25] Farg MA, Konopka A, Soo KY, Ito D, Atkin JD. The DNA damage response (DDR) is induced by the C9orf72 repeat expansion in amyotrophic lateral sclerosis. Human Molecular Genetics. 2017;**26**:2882-2896. DOI: 10.1093/hmg/ddx170

[26] Lopez-Gonzalez R, Lu Y, Gendron TF, Karydas A, Tran H, Yang D, et al. Poly(GR) in C9ORF72 - related ALS/FTD compromises mitochondrial function and increases oxidative stress and DNA damage in iPSC-derived motor neurons. Neuron. 2016;**92**:383-391. DOI: 10.1016/j.neuron.2016.09.015

[27] Sariki SK, Sahu PK, Golla U, Singh V, Azad GK, Tomar RS. Sen1, the homolog of human Senataxin, is critical for cell survival through regulation of redox homeostasis, mitochondrial function, and the TOR pathway in *Saccharomyces cerevisiae*. The FEBS Journal. 2016;**283**:4056-4083. DOI: 10.1111/febs.13917

[28] Sama RRK, Ward CL, Bosco DA. Functions of FUS/TLS from DNA repair to stress response: Implications for ALS. ASN Neuro. 2014;**6**:175909141454447. DOI: 10.1177/1759091414544472

[29] Walker C, El-Khamisy SF. Perturbed autophagy and DNA repair converge to promote neurodegeneration in amyotrophic lateral sclerosis and dementia. Brain. 2018;**141**:1247-1262. DOI: 10.1093/brain/awy076

[30] Browne SE, Yang L, DiMauro J-P, Fuller SW, Licata SC, Beal MF. Bioenergetic abnormalities in discrete cerebral motor pathways presage spinal cord pathology in the G93A SOD1 mouse model of ALS. Neurobiology of Disease. 2006;**22**:599-610. DOI: 10.1016/j.nbd.2006.01.001

[31] Mattiazzi M, D'Aurelio M, Gajewski CD, Martushova K, Kiaei M, Beal MF, et al. Mutated human SOD1 causes dysfunction of oxidative phosphorylation in mitochondria of transgenic mice. The Journal of Biological Chemistry. 2002;**277**:29626-29633. DOI: 10.1074/jbc.M203065200

[32] Faes L, Callewaert G. Mitochondrial dysfunction in familial amyotrophic lateral sclerosis. Journal of Bioenergetics and Biomembranes. 2011;**43**:587-592. DOI: 10.1007/s10863-011-9393-0

[33] Coussee E, De Smet P, Bogaert E, Elens I, Van Damme P, Willems P, et al. G37R SOD1 mutant alters mitochondrial complex I activity, Ca^{2+} uptake and ATP production. Cell Calcium. 2011;**49**:217-225. DOI: 10.1016/j.ceca.2011.02.004

[34] Tradewell ML, Cooper LA, Minotti S, Durham HD. Calcium dysregulation, mitochondrial pathology and protein aggregation in a culture model of amyotrophic lateral sclerosis: Mechanistic relationship and differential sensitivity to intervention. Neurobiology of Disease. 2011;**42**:265-275. DOI: 10.1016/j.nbd.2011.01.016

[35] Jaiswal MK, Keller BU. Cu/Zn superoxide dismutase typical for familial amyotrophic lateral sclerosis increases the vulnerability of mitochondria and perturbs Ca^{2+} homeostasis in SOD1 ^{G93A} mice. Molecular Pharmacology. 2009;**75**:478-489. DOI: 10.1124/mol.108.050831

[36] Hu C, Huang Y, Li L. Drp1-dependent mitochondrial fission plays critical roles in physiological and pathological progresses in mammals. IJMS. 2017;**18**:144. DOI: 10.3390/ijms18010144

[37] Joshi AU, Saw NL, Vogel H, Cunnigham AD, Shamloo M, Mochly-Rosen D. Inhibition of Drp1/Fis1 interaction slows progression of amyotrophic lateral sclerosis. EMBO Molecular Medicine. 2018;**10**. DOI: 10.15252/emmm.201708166

[38] Babbar M, Sheikh MS. Metabolic stress and disorders related to alterations in mitochondrial fission or fusion. Molecular and Cellular Pharmacology. 2013;**5**:109-133

[39] Kong J, Xu Z. Massive mitochondrial degeneration in motor neurons triggers the onset of amyotrophic lateral sclerosis in mice expressing a mutant SOD1. The Journal of Neuroscience. 1998;**18**:3241-3250

[40] Magrané J, Cortez C, Gan W-B, Manfredi G. Abnormal mitochondrial transport and morphology are common pathological denominators in SOD1 and TDP-43 ALS mouse models. Human Molecular Genetics. 2014;**23**:1413-1424. DOI: 10.1093/hmg/ddt528

[41] Vande Velde C, McDonald KK, Boukhedimi Y, McAlonis-Downes M, Lobsiger CS, Bel Hadj S, et al. Misfolded SOD1 associated with motor neuron mitochondria alters mitochondrial shape and distribution prior to clinical onset. PLoS One. 2011;**6**:e22031. DOI: 10.1371/journal.pone.0022031

[42] Nakaya T, Maragkakis M. Amyotrophic lateral sclerosis associated FUS mutation shortens mitochondria and induces neurotoxicity. Scientific

Reports. 2018;**8**:15575. DOI: 10.1038/s41598-018-33964-0

[43] Deng J, Yang M, Chen Y, Chen X, Liu J, Sun S, et al. FUS interacts with HSP60 to promote mitochondrial damage. PLoS Genetics. 2015;**11**:e1005357. DOI: 10.1371/journal.pgen.1005357

[44] Hansen JJ, Dürr A, Cournu-Rebeix I, Georgopoulos C, Ang D, Nielsen MN, et al. Hereditary spastic paraplegia SPG13 is associated with a mutation in the gene encoding the mitochondrial chaperonin Hsp60. American Journal of Human Genetics. 2002;**70**:1328-1332. DOI: 10.1086/339935

[45] Deng J, Wang P, Chen X, Cheng H, Liu J, Fushimi K, et al. FUS interacts with ATP synthase beta subunit and induces mitochondrial unfolded protein response in cellular and animal models. Proceedings of the National Academy of Sciences of the United States of America. 2018;**115**:E9678-E9686. DOI: 10.1073/pnas.1806655115

[46] Wang W, Wang L, Lu J, Siedlak SL, Fujioka H, Liang J, et al. The inhibition of TDP-43 mitochondrial localization blocks its neuronal toxicity. Nature Medicine. 2016;**22**:869-878. DOI: 10.1038/nm.4130

[47] Stoica R, Paillusson S, Gomez-Suaga P, Mitchell JC, Lau DH, Gray EH, et al. ALS/FTD-associated FUS activates GSK-3β to disrupt the VAPB-PTPIP51 interaction and ER-mitochondria associations. EMBO Reports. 2016;**17**:1326-1342. DOI: 10.15252/embr.201541726

[48] Yang J-L, Weissman L, Bohr VA, Mattson MP. Mitochondrial DNA damage and repair in neurodegenerative disorders. DNA Repair. 2008;**7**:1110-1120. DOI: 10.1016/j.dnarep.2008.03.012

[49] Bermúdez-Guzmán L, Leal A. DNA repair deficiency in neuropathogenesis: When all roads lead to mitochondria. Translational Neurodegeneration. 2019;**8**:14. DOI: 10.1186/s40035-019-0156-x

[50] Alencar RR, Batalha CMPF, Freire TS, de Souza-Pinto NC. Enzymology of mitochondrial DNA repair. In: The Enzymes. Elsevier; 2019. p. S1874604719300022. DOI: 10.1016/bs.enz.2019.06.002

[51] Murakami T, Nagai M, Miyazaki K, Morimoto N, Ohta Y, Kurata T, et al. Early decrease of mitochondrial DNA repair enzymes in spinal motor neurons of presymptomatic transgenic mice carrying a mutant SOD1 gene. Brain Research. 2007;**1150**:182-189. DOI: 10.1016/j.brainres.2007.02.057

[52] Dhaliwal GK, Grewal RP. Mitochondrial DNA deletion mutation levels are elevated in ALS brains. Neuroreport. 2000;**11**:2507-2509. DOI: 10.1097/00001756-200008030-00032

[53] Kikuchi H, Furuta A, Nishioka K, Suzuki S, Nakabeppu Y, Iwaki T. Impairment of mitochondrial DNA repair enzymes against accumulation of 8-oxo-guanine in the spinal motor neurons of amyotrophic lateral sclerosis. Acta Neuropathologica. 2002;**103**:408-414. DOI: 10.1007/s00401-001-0480-x

[54] Martin LJ, Liu Z, Chen K, Price AC, Pan Y, Swaby JA, et al. Motor neuron degeneration in amyotrophic lateral sclerosis mutant superoxide dismutase-1 transgenic mice: Mechanisms of mitochondriopathy and cell death. The Journal of Comparative Neurology. 2007;**500**:20-46. DOI: 10.1002/cne.21160

[55] Ray Chaudhuri A, Nussenzweig A. The multifaceted roles of PARP1 in DNA repair and chromatin remodelling. Nature Reviews. Molecular Cell Biology. 2017;**18**:610-621. DOI: 10.1038/nrm.2017.53

[56] Hoch NC, Hanzlikova H, Rulten SL, Tétreault M, Komulainen E, Ju L, et al. XRCC1 mutation is associated with PARP1 hyperactivation and cerebellar ataxia. Nature. 2017;**541**:87-91. DOI: 10.1038/nature20790

[57] Rulten SL, Rotheray A, Green RL, Grundy GJ, Moore DAQ, Gómez-Herreros F, et al. PARP-1 dependent recruitment of the amyotrophic lateral sclerosis-associated protein FUS/TLS to sites of oxidative DNA damage. Nucleic Acids Research. 2014;**42**:307-314. DOI: 10.1093/nar/gkt835

[58] Martire S, Mosca L, d'Erme M. PARP-1 involvement in neurodegeneration: A focus on Alzheimer's and Parkinson's diseases. Mechanisms of Ageing and Development. 2015;**146-148**:53-64. DOI: 10.1016/j.mad.2015.04.001

[59] Narne P, Pandey V, Simhadri PK, Phanithi PB. Poly(ADP-ribose) polymerase-1 hyperactivation in neurodegenerative diseases: The death knell tolls for neurons. Seminars in Cell and Developmental Biology. 2017;**63**:154-166. DOI: 10.1016/j.semcdb.2016.11.007

[60] Ramadori G, Lee CE, Bookout AL, Lee S, Williams KW, Anderson J, et al. Brain SIRT1: Anatomical distribution and regulation by energy availability. Journal of Neuroscience. 2008;**28**:9989-9996. DOI: 10.1523/JNEUROSCI.3257-08.2008

[61] Cantó C, Menzies KJ, Auwerx J. NAD+ metabolism and the control of energy homeostasis: A balancing act between mitochondria and the nucleus. Cell Metabolism. 2015;**22**:31-53. DOI: 10.1016/j.cmet.2015.05.023

[62] Scheibye-Knudsen M, Mitchell SJ, Fang EF, Iyama T, Ward T, Wang J, et al. A high-fat diet and NAD + activate Sirt1 to rescue premature aging in Cockayne syndrome. Cell Metabolism. 2014;**20**:840-855. DOI: 10.1016/j.cmet.2014.10.005

[63] Bai P, Cantó C, Oudart H, Brunyánszki A, Cen Y, Thomas C, et al. PARP-1 inhibition increases mitochondrial metabolism through SIRT1 activation. Cell Metabolism. 2011;**13**:461-468. DOI: 10.1016/j.cmet.2011.03.004

[64] Yu J, Auwerx J. The role of Sirtuins in the control of metabolic homeostasis. Annals of the New York Academy of Sciences. 2009;**1173**:E10-E19. DOI: 10.1111/j.1749-6632.2009.04952.x

[65] Nemoto S, Fergusson MM, Finkel T. SIRT1 functionally interacts with the metabolic regulator and transcriptional coactivator PGC-1α. The Journal of Biological Chemistry. 2005;**280**:16456-16460. DOI: 10.1074/jbc.M501485200

[66] St-Pierre J, Drori S, Uldry M, Silvaggi JM, Rhee J, Jäger S, et al. Suppression of reactive oxygen species and neurodegeneration by the PGC-1 transcriptional coactivators. Cell. 2006;**127**:397-408. DOI: 10.1016/j.cell.2006.09.024

[67] Xu J, Jackson CW, Khoury N, Escobar I, Perez-Pinzon MA. Brain SIRT1 mediates metabolic homeostasis and neuroprotection. Frontiers in Endocrinology. 2018;**9**:702. DOI: 10.3389/fendo.2018.00702

[68] Aquilano K, Vigilanza P, Baldelli S, Pagliei B, Rotilio G, Ciriolo MR. Peroxisome proliferator-activated receptor γ co-activator 1α (PGC-1α) and Sirtuin 1 (SIRT1) reside in mitochondria: Possible direct function in mitochondrial biogenesis. The Journal of Biological Chemistry. 2010;**285**:21590-21599. DOI: 10.1074/jbc.M109.070169

[69] Fanibunda SE, Deb S, Maniyadath B, Tiwari P, Ghai U,

Gupta S, et al. Serotonin regulates mitochondrial biogenesis and function in rodent cortical neurons via the 5-HT2A receptor and SIRT1–PGC-1α axis. Proceedings of the National Academy of Sciences of the United States of America. 2019;**116**:11028-11037. DOI: 10.1073/pnas.1821332116

[70] Brunet A. Stress-dependent regulation of FOXO transcription factors by the SIRT1 deacetylase. Science. 2004;**303**:2011-2015. DOI: 10.1126/science.1094637

[71] Cantó C, Gerhart-Hines Z, Feige JN, Lagouge M, Noriega L, Milne JC, et al. AMPK regulates energy expenditure by modulating NAD+ metabolism and SIRT1 activity. Nature. 2009;**458**:1056-1060. DOI: 10.1038/nature07813

[72] Tang BL. Sirt1 and the mitochondria. Molecules and Cells. 2016;**39**:87-95. DOI: 10.14348/MOLCELLS.2016.2318

[73] Fang EF, Scheibye-Knudsen M, Brace LE, Kassahun H, SenGupta T, Nilsen H, et al. Defective mitophagy in XPA via PARP-1 hyperactivation and NAD+/SIRT1 reduction. Cell. 2014;**157**:882-896. DOI: 10.1016/j.cell.2014.03.026

[74] Mouchiroud L, Houtkooper RH, Moullan N, Katsyuba E, Ryu D, Cantó C, et al. The NAD+/Sirtuin pathway modulates longevity through activation of mitochondrial UPR and FOXO signaling. Cell. 2013;**154**:430-441. DOI: 10.1016/j.cell.2013.06.016

[75] Wang X, Zhang Q, Bao R, Zhang N, Wang Y, Polo-Parada L, et al. Deletion of nampt in projection neurons of adult mice leads to motor dysfunction, neurodegeneration, and death. Cell Reports. 2017;**20**:2184-2200. DOI: 10.1016/j.celrep.2017.08.022

[76] Price NL, Gomes AP, Ling AJY, Duarte FV, Martin-Montalvo A, North BJ, et al. SIRT1 is required for AMPK activation and the beneficial effects of resveratrol on mitochondrial function. Cell Metabolism. 2012;**15**:675-690. DOI: 10.1016/j.cmet.2012.04.003

[77] Kim D, Nguyen MD, Dobbin MM, Fischer A, Sananbenesi F, Rodgers JT, et al. SIRT1 deacetylase protects against neurodegeneration in models for Alzheimer's disease and amyotrophic lateral sclerosis. The EMBO Journal. 2007;**26**:3169-3179. DOI: 10.1038/sj.emboj.7601758

[78] Dobbin MM, Madabhushi R, Pan L, Chen Y, Kim D, Gao J, et al. SIRT1 collaborates with ATM and HDAC1 to maintain genomic stability in neurons. Nature Neuroscience. 2013;**16**:1008-1015. DOI: 10.1038/nn.3460

[79] Jeong J, Juhn K, Lee H, Kim S-H, Min B-H, Lee K-M, et al. SIRT1 promotes DNA repair activity and deacetylation of Ku70. Experimental and Molecular Medicine. 2007;**39**:8-13. DOI: 10.1038/emm.2007.2

[80] Li K, Casta A, Wang R, Lozada E, Fan W, Kane S, et al. Regulation of WRN protein cellular localization and enzymatic activities by SIRT1-mediated deacetylation. The Journal of Biological Chemistry. 2008;**283**:7590-7598. DOI: 10.1074/jbc.M709707200

[81] Yuan Z, Zhang X, Sengupta N, Lane WS, Seto E. SIRT1 regulates the function of the Nijmegen breakage syndrome protein. Molecular Cell. 2007;**27**:149-162. DOI: 10.1016/j.molcel.2007.05.029

[82] Yamamori T, DeRicco J, Naqvi A, Hoffman TA, Mattagajasingh I, Kasuno K, et al. SIRT1 deacetylates APE1 and regulates cellular base excision repair. Nucleic Acids Research. 2010;**38**:832-845. DOI: 10.1093/nar/gkp1039

[83] Madabushi A, Hwang B-J, Jin J, Lu A-L. Histone deacetylase SIRT1 modulates and deacetylates DNA base excision repair enzyme thymine DNA glycosylase. The Biochemical Journal. 2013;**456**:89-98. DOI: 10.1042/BJ20130670

[84] Fan W, Luo J. SIRT1 regulates UV-induced DNA repair through deacetylating XPA. Molecular Cell. 2010;**39**:247-258. DOI: 10.1016/j.molcel.2010.07.006

[85] Wang W-Y, Pan L, Su SC, Quinn EJ, Sasaki M, Jimenez JC, et al. Interaction of FUS and HDAC1 regulates DNA damage response and repair in neurons. Nature Neuroscience. 2013;**16**:1383-1391. DOI: 10.1038/nn.3514

[86] Higelin J, Demestre M, Putz S, Delling JP, Jacob C, Lutz A-K, et al. FUS mislocalization and vulnerability to DNA damage in ALS patients derived hiPSCs and aging motoneurons. Frontiers in Cellular Neuroscience. 2016;**10**. DOI: 10.3389/fncel.2016.00290

[87] Wang H, Hegde ML. New mechanisms of DNA repair defects in fused in sarcoma–associated neurodegeneration: Stage set for DNA repair-based therapeutics? Journal of Experimental Neuroscience. 2019;**13**:117906951985635. DOI: 10.1177/1179069519856358

[88] Wang H, Guo W, Mitra J, Hegde PM, Vandoorne T, Eckelmann BJ, et al. Mutant FUS causes DNA ligation defects to inhibit oxidative damage repair in amyotrophic lateral sclerosis. Nature Communications. 2018;**9**:3683. DOI: 10.1038/s41467-018-06111-6

[89] Gao Y, Katyal S, Lee Y, Zhao J, Rehg JE, Russell HR, et al. DNA ligase III is critical for mtDNA integrity but not Xrcc1-mediated nuclear DNA repair. Nature. 2011;**471**:240-244. DOI: 10.1038/nature09773

[90] Geisler S, Holmström KM, Skujat D, Fiesel FC, Rothfuss OC, Kahle PJ, et al. PINK1/Parkin-mediated mitophagy is dependent on VDAC1 and p62/SQSTM1. Nature Cell Biology. 2010;**12**:119-131. DOI: 10.1038/ncb2012

[91] Ding W-X, Ni H-M, Li M, Liao Y, Chen X, Stolz DB, et al. Nix is critical to two distinct phases of mitophagy, reactive oxygen species-mediated autophagy induction and Parkin-ubiquitin-p62-mediated mitochondrial priming. The Journal of Biological Chemistry. 2010;**285**:27879-27890. DOI: 10.1074/jbc.M110.119537

[92] Liu H, Dai C, Fan Y, Guo B, Ren K, Sun T, et al. From autophagy to mitophagy: The roles of P62 in neurodegenerative diseases. Journal of Bioenergetics and Biomembranes. 2017;**49**:413-422. DOI: 10.1007/s10863-017-9727-7

[93] Karabiyik C, Lee MJ, Rubinsztein DC. Autophagy impairment in Parkinson's disease. Essays in Biochemistry. 2017;**61**:711-720. DOI: 10.1042/EBC20170023

[94] Sato S, Uchihara T, Fukuda T, Noda S, Kondo H, Saiki S, et al. Loss of autophagy in dopaminergic neurons causes Lewy pathology and motor dysfunction in aged mice. Scientific Reports. 2018;**8**:2813. DOI: 10.1038/s41598-018-21325-w

[95] Wong YC, Holzbaur ELF. Optineurin is an autophagy receptor for damaged mitochondria in parkin-mediated mitophagy that is disrupted by an ALS-linked mutation. Proceedings of the National Academy of Sciences of the United States of America. 2014;**111**:E4439-E4448. DOI: 10.1073/pnas.1405752111

[96] Fang EF, Hou Y, Palikaras K, Adriaanse BA, Kerr JS, Yang B, et al. Mitophagy inhibits amyloid-β and tau pathology and reverses cognitive deficits

in models of Alzheimer's disease. Nature Neuroscience. 2019;**22**:401-412. DOI: 10.1038/s41593-018-0332-9

[97] Wang Y, Zhang N, Zhang L, Li R, Fu W, Ma K, et al. Autophagy regulates chromatin ubiquitination in DNA damage response through elimination of SQSTM1/p62. Molecular Cell. 2016;**63**:34-48. DOI: 10.1016/j.molcel.2016.05.027

[98] Chang C-Y, Liang M-Z, Chen L. Current progress of mitochondrial transplantation that promotes neuronal regeneration. Translational Neurodegeneration. 2019;**8**:17. DOI: 10.1186/s40035-019-0158-8

[99] Hayakawa K, Esposito E, Wang X, Terasaki Y, Liu Y, Xing C, et al. Transfer of mitochondria from astrocytes to neurons after stroke. Nature. 2016;**535**:551-555. DOI: 10.1038/nature18928

[100] McCully JD, Levitsky S, del Nido PJ, Cowan DB. Mitochondrial transplantation for therapeutic use. Clinical and Translational Medicine. 2016;**5**:16. DOI: 10.1186/s40169-016-0095-4

[101] Masuzawa A, Black KM, Pacak CA, Ericsson M, Barnett RJ, Drumm C, et al. Transplantation of autologously derived mitochondria protects the heart from ischemia-reperfusion injury. American Journal of Physiology. Heart and Circulatory Physiology. 2013;**304**:H966-H982. DOI: 10.1152/ajpheart.00883.2012

[102] Shi X, Zhao M, Fu C, Fu A. Intravenous administration of mitochondria for treating experimental Parkinson's disease. Mitochondrion. 2017;**34**:91-100. DOI: 10.1016/j.mito.2017.02.005

[103] Wilkins MH, Morris KJ. New therapeutics to modulate mitochondrial function in neurodegenerative disorders. Current Pharmaceutical Design. 2017;**23**:731-752. DOI: 10.2174/1381612822666161230144517

Section 2

Emerging Etiopathology and Implications

Chapter 5

The Role of Extracellular Vesicles in the Progression of ALS and Their Potential as Biomarkers and Therapeutic Agents with Which to Combat the Disease

Changho Chun, Alec S.T. Smith, Mark Bothwell and David L. Mack

Abstract

Amyotrophic lateral sclerosis (ALS) is a fatal neurodegenerative disease that impairs motor neuron function, leading to severe muscular atrophy. The non-cell autonomous and heterogeneous nature of the disease has so far hindered attempts to define ALS etiology, leaving the disease incurable and without effective treatments. Recent studies have focused on the pathologic role of intercellular communication between nerve cells to further our understanding of ALS pathophysiology. In this chapter, we summarize recent works investigating the role of extracellular vesicles (EVs) as a means of cellular crosstalk for ALS disease propagation, diagnosis, and treatment. There is growing evidence that EVs secreted by the majority of mammalian cells serve as effective biomolecule carriers to modulate recipient cell behavior. This underscores the need to understand the EV-mediated interplay that occurs within irreversibly degenerating nervous tissue in ALS patients. Additionally, we highlight current gaps in EV-ALS research, especially in terms of the pathologic role and responsibilities of specific EV cargos in diseased cells, specificity issues associated with the use of EVs in ALS diagnosis, and the efficacy of EV-mediated treatments for the restoration of diseased neuromuscular tissue. Finally, we provide suggestions for future EV-ALS research to better understand, diagnose, and cure this inveterate disease.

Keywords: ALS, extracellular vesicle, exosome, propagation, biomarker, therapeutic agent

1. Introduction

Amyotrophic Lateral Sclerosis (ALS), also known as Lou Gehrig's disease, is a heterogeneous neurodegenerative disease that primarily impairs both upper and lower motor neurons [1, 2]. 5000 people in the United States are diagnosed with ALS each year, mostly between the ages of 40 and 70. The irreversibly progressive nature of ALS leads to the death of most patients within 2–5 years of diagnosis, typically due to respiratory failure [1, 3]. In most patients, the cause of ALS is unknown. Only 10% of patients have a familial history of ALS, caused by specific mutations in their genomes, while 90% are exhibit sporadic ALS due to unknown causal factors [1, 4, 5]. The lack of understanding concerning ALS disease mechanisms has led to the development of very few FDA approved drugs. To date, those drugs that have progressed to the US market merely slow down disease progression by a few months and do little to restore patient's neuromuscular function [6]. As progressive degeneration and the non-cell autonomous nature of ALS are known to be major reasons for this stalemate, the aim of much current ALS research is focused on understanding the diverse interplay between neurons and non-neuronal components in neuromuscular tissue. Among the non-neuronal components, glial cells and their crosstalk with neurons have been major targets of study regarding symptomatic development and progression in ALS [7–10]. Accordingly, research into a myriad of proteins and RNAs known to be transmissible between neurons and glial cells has been gaining interest in recent years. It is already well-established that such agents can act as molecular 'messengers' to alter the behavior of nearby cells in ALS, but the detailed mechanisms that underpin specific cargo selection, initiation of transport, and subsequent activation of the internalized biomolecules are not fully understood.

Extracellular vesicles (EVs) are lipid bi-layered particles, less than 2 μm in size, secreted by the majority of mammalian cells, including nerve cells, to mediate diverse paracrine signaling pathways [11–13]. These vesicles are typically classified into three categories: microvesicles, apoptotic bodies, and exosomes [14]. Microvesicles and apoptotic bodies are normally 0.1–2 μm in size and bud directly from the plasma membrane. Exosomes, on the other hand, are smaller (50–150 nm) and are generated within cytoplasmic multivesicular bodies (MVBs) before being secreted to the extracellular space through subsequent fusion of MVBs with the plasma membrane [11, 15].

In many neurodegenerative disorders, EVs derived from nerve cells have been proposed to be responsible for spreading neurotoxins to normal cells, accelerating disease progression [16–20]. In the diseased cell, misregulated proteins serve as 'templates' for subsequent protein oligomerization, generating insoluble toxic aggregates. Such aggregates are then either degraded by lysosomes using a 'self-clearance' mechanism, or incorporated into MVBs and/or the plasma membrane facilitating subsequent release into the extracellular space [21]. EV-loaded biomolecules can then be transmitted to recipient cells primarily by endocytosis but also by endosomal fusion of the EV membrane with cell's plasma membrane [22]. For example, exosomes facilitate the intercellular delivery of amyloid beta (Aβ) peptides in Alzheimer's disease, leading to plaque formation in the recipient cells [19, 20]. A similar trend of EV-mediated or free protein spreading in a 'prion-like' manner is observed in Parkinson's disease (PD). Specifically, studies with mice have demonstrated that grafted cells containing aggregated α-synuclein can transfer these protein aggregates to healthy brain tissue [23].

As the contents of EVs reflect the physiological status of the original cell, recent studies have begun to evaluate the possibility of using these structures as biomarkers with which to gauge the onset and progression of a diverse range of neurodegenerative diseases. Issues remain with identifying tissue specificity and cell type of origin for pathogenic EVs found in body fluids. However, convenient sampling and improved understanding of internal cargo molecules' function has led to EV's being seen as one of the strongest candidate classes for next generation prognosis/diagnosis screening. As with other degenerative diseases of the central nervous system (CNS), much recent work on ALS has focused on investigating the pathological role of EVs in diseased neuromuscular tissue, as well as evaluating their applicability in the early diagnosis and further treatment of the disease. In this review, we will highlight recent research studying the diverse roles of EVs in ALS progression, diagnosis, and treatment. In addition, we will discuss possible solutions for unsolved problems in this area and suggest future directions for ALS-EV research to further our understanding of ALS pathology and help develop advanced diagnosis and treatment methods using EVs.

2. EVs as dysregulated biomolecule carriers for disease propagation in ALS

ALS tissues commonly contain cells supporting dysregulated protein aggregates in their cytoplasm and these structures often exert detrimental effects on cell viability and function. SOD1 (superoxide dismutase 1) and TDP-43 (transactive DNA binding protein 43 kDa), encoded by the *SOD1* and *TARDBP* genes respectively, are the most well-studied proteins susceptible to ALS-associated aggregation. Aggregation of these proteins, in some cases due to destabilizing mutations, are known to be actively involved in motor neuron degeneration in both familial and sporadic ALS [1, 24, 25]. The SOD1 enzyme resides in the cytoplasm of normal cells to regulate oxidative stress by converting free superoxide radicals into molecular oxygen [2]. There are more than 180 mutations reported in the *SOD1* gene, and oligomerization of the encoded proteins has been shown to cause increased intracellular oxidative stress and anomalous metal binding [2]. However, the pathologic pathway connecting *SOD1* mutation, protein dysregulation, and subsequent neurodegeneration have yet to be defined in a comprehensive manner [2, 26]. TDP-43 is a highly conserved nuclear RNA and DNA binding protein, known to be involved in transcriptomic regulation, primarily by RNA splicing but also by effects on mRNA transport and stability, effects on microRNA production, and participating in DNA repair [27–31]. Approximately 97% of ALS patients have abnormally aggregated TDP-43 in their neurons, even without direct mutation of the *TARDBP* gene, leading to ALS proteinopathic characteristics in their pathology [6, 32].

Strikingly, recent ALS studies have demonstrated that abnormally transformed proteins, such as SOD1 and TDP-43, do not merely impair the cells of origin, but migrate to neighboring cells by means of extracellular exosome release, resulting in a spread of their cytotoxic effect to recipient cells [33, 34]. Exosome shuttling has been shown to be a preferred cellular mechanism for removing intracellular toxic molecules to the extracellular space [35]. The exosomal loading of cytotoxic protein aggregates is beneficial to host cells since it minimizes the physiological damage caused by these structures. Such phenomena could be promoted by the host cell recognizing an increase in intracellular protein aggregation or impaired lysosomal autophagy. Interestingly, normal neurons cultured with TDP-43 aggregate-loaded exosomes induce cytoplasmic redistribution of endogenous TDP-43, leading to an exacerbation of the disease phenotype in mice [36]. Moreover, proteins packaged in extracellular vesicles are preferentially taken up by recipient cells and exhibit a greater detrimental physiological effect compared to free protein release, highlighting a crucial role for EV and plasma membrane tethered proteins in regulating protein internalization and functional activation [37]. These studies suggest an important interaction between exogenous TDP-43 transported via extracellular vesicles and endogenous TDP-43 expressed by the recipient cell. Such interactions constitute a pre-requisite for 'prion-like' seeding followed by cytoplasmic protein redistribution and offer a potential mechanism for the rapid propagation of disease phenotypes throughout the motor neuron pool. Indeed, when insoluble TDP-43 aggregates taken from ALS brain were introduced to neuron-like SH-SY5Y cells endogenously expressing normal TDP-43, the treatment induced significant aggregation of TDP-43 in recipient cells in a self-templating manner [38]. Similarly, SOD1 aggregates transferred via exosomes have been shown to work as self-templating 'seeds' in recipient cells, leading to the propagation of a misfolded protein that persists in culture over multiple passages and population doublings [34].

Although recent studies have observed intercellular protein transmission via EVs, their specific roles in neuromuscular pathophysiology are poorly understood. In particular, how the transfer of abnormal proteins induces subsequent neuronal damage and a breakdown in their electrophysiological function has yet to be elucidated. Furthermore, by taking into account that ALS exhibits non-neuron autonomous characteristics, it is essential to obtain a more comprehensive understanding of whether and how non-neuronal nerve cells can damage neuromuscular function via the exosomal transfer pathway. **Table 1** provides an overview of the studies performed so far relating to the role of EVs in propagating ALS pathologies to neighboring cells and these studies are discussed in more detail throughout this section.

Among non-neuronal cell types, astrocytes have gained significant interest as carriers of detrimental protein aggregates in ALS tissues. Secretome analysis of astrocytic exosomes from SOD1 (G93A) mutant mice were reported to contain SOD1 aggregates, and the exosomal release of these structures accounted for a larger proportion of SOD1 transport than free SOD1 release [4, 14]. In addition, proteomic analysis has revealed that proteins involved in vesicle trafficking are downregulated in mutant astrocytes, indicating a possible impairment of protein disposal in ALS astrocytes. Moreover, wild-type mice transplanted with astrocyte progenitors expressing mutant SOD1 exhibit motor neuron impairment, raising the reasonable postulation that diseased astrocytes utilize extracellular vesicle-mediated paracrine communication to deliver pathogenic protein aggregates to motor neurons [4, 14]. Another quantitative proteomic analysis of EVs derived from ALS nervous tissue showed a relative absence of the microglial marker (CD11b) but positive expression for the astrocyte marker (GLAST) and the synaptic marker (SNAP25), indicating that astrocytes and neurons may constitute the major cell types involved in EV-mediated communication in the CNS [7]. However, as the main function of microglia in the CNS is immune response regulation under pro-inflammatory conditions, microglia might also actively secrete EVs within an immune-active environment to modulate the immune response of other nerve cells. Since ALS is reported to have autoimmune disease characteristics as well [39, 40], a pathogenic role for EVs secreted from diseased microglia in ALS tissue could be another important subject to explore.

Do skeletal muscle cells also secrete EVs for neuronal uptake? The breakdown of neuromuscular junctions (NMJs; the synapses connecting lower motor neurons and skeletal muscle fibers) is a critical early indicator of pathological onset in ALS. However, it remains unclear whether NMJ breakdown occurs due to general ill health of the motor neuron or some aberrant signaling between these neurons and their afferent synaptic contacts. If the latter is true, a reasonable hypothesis would be that ALS progression is affected by paracrine communication between skeletal muscle and motor neurons. To this point, an interesting study in 2017 described the involvement of skeletal muscle in EV-based crosstalk in neuromuscular tissues. In ALS muscle biopsies, noticeable accumulation of MVBs containing exosome-like vesicles were measured, with significant increases in vesicular protein concentrations reported when compared with controls. In addition to the denser protein accumulation reported in the EVs, ALS skeletal muscle-derived EVs were shown to exclusively damage neuronal viability *in vitro* [4, 14].

Role of EV	Study method	Source of EV	Significance	Unknowns	Reference
Dysregulated protein and RNA carrier	*In vitro* study with astrocytes and mouse motor neurons	Directly differentiated astrocytes from fALS (C9ORF72) patient-derived fibroblast	Micro-RNAs in ALS astrocyte-derived extracellular vesicle (EV) caused neuronal network degeneration and growth cone impairment	The role of C9ORF72 protein for dysregulated miRNA encapsulation in EV	Varcianna et al. [41]
	In vitro/ex vivo study for whole tissue vesicle isolation	Brain- and spinal cord tissue from NTg and SOD1 mutant mice	Brain-derived astrocytes and neurons, but not microglia, were the main EV source in CNS	Detailed cargo modification pattern of EVs in the diseased cells	Silverman et al. [7]
	Clinical research with sporadic ALS patients' body fluid for EV analysis	Venous blood of sALS patients	Microvesicles of ALS patients were enriched with potentially pathological protein (SOD1, TDP-43, FUS), while exosomes did not show any protein changes	Contradictory result with other (*in vitro*) studies that suggested huge loading of dysregulated proteins in exosomes of ALS mutant cells	Sproviero et al. [59]
	In vitro study with ALS mouse muscle-derived exosomes treated to primary/iPSC-derived motor neurons	Skeletal muscle cells from SOD1 mutant mouse	EVs derived from ALS myotubes encapsulated H2-AX (neurotoxin) which suggests possible dissemination of various neurotoxic molecules from diseased skeletal muscle to normal neurons	Is H2-AX a major neurotoxin in human ALS skeletal muscle as well?	Gall et al. [60]
	In vitro study using Neuro2a and primary neurons to study the role of exosomes in ALS proteinopathy	Primary neurons and Neuro2a cells from ALS mouse brain	Exosome secretion was beneficial in neuronal clearance of pathological TDP-43, but also it might be responsible for the propagation of the toxic TDP-43 aggregates to the other cells	Should we inhibit exosome secretion to prevent aggregated TDP-43 propagation or promote the secretion for TDP-43 clearance in neurons?	Iguchi et al. [36]
	In vitro co-culture of NSC-34 with cortical	Mutant DPR (dipeptide repeat proteins)	DPRs can be transmitted to neurons and glial cells with/	Difference between propagated DPRs and other	Westergard et al. [61]

Role of EV	Study method	Source of EV	Significance	Unknowns	Reference
	neurons and astrocytes	transfected NSC-34 cells	without exosome involvement	dysregulated proteins (TDP-43, SOD1) in terms of their neurodegeneration effect?	
	In vitro study using ALS patient-derived exosomes and human glioma cell line (U251)	CSF from 18 sALS patients	ALS-CSF incubation with U251 cells increased mis-located TDP-43 in the glioma cells and induced their apoptotic behavior and macro autophagy process	Connection between propagated TDP-43 and autophagy mechanism in recipient cells	Zhou et al. [62]
	In vitro study using primary neurons and TDP-43 transfected HEK cells	ALS post-mortem lysate, primary cortical mouse neurons and HEK cells	TDP-43 oligomers were present in EVs and showed that microvesicular TDP-43 exerts higher toxicity than free TDP-43	EV encapsulating pathway of neurotoxic TDP-43 oligomers	Feiler et al. [37]
	In vitro study with neuroblastoma cells with brain tissue obtained from ALS/FTD patients	Neuroblastoma cells expressing TDP-43 and SOD1	Misfolded wild-type proteins could traverse cell-to-cell as a self-templating 'seed' either as free protein aggregates or loaded on the surface of exosomes	Which specific receptors control the uptake of misfolded TDP-43/ SOD1 presented on exosomes?	Nonaka et al. [38]
	In vitro study analyzing neurotoxic effect and amount of SOD1 protein encapsulated in astrocytic exosomes	Primary astrocytes from mouse expressing human mutant SOD1	Mutant SOD1 astrocytes released increased number of exosomes, which were toxic for motor neurons	Protein factors which involved in mutant SOD1 astrocytic exosome	Basso et al. [26]

Table 1.
Overview of the recent findings regarding roles for extracellular vesicles in ALS disease propagation.

Although dysregulated protein transfer is of major interest in ALS-EV research, the role of transmissible miRNAs in facilitating ALS progression should not be overlooked. EVs obtained from astrocytes derived from ALS patient post-mortem tissue (*C9ORF72* mutation) have been shown to display a neurotoxic phenotype, inducing mouse motor neuron degeneration, though fewer EVs were secreted from diseased astrocytes than normal controls [41]. Dysregulated miR-494-3p was identified as a main component of the diseased EVs. This astrocyte-specific miRNA is known to negatively regulate semaphorin-3A expression, which is highly involved in axonal growth and maintenance [41]. Similarly, exosomes secreted by mouse-derived motor neuron-like cells (NSC-34) transfected with a human SOD1 mutant variant were enriched with miR-124. This miRNA was in turn transmissible to the microglia, where it induced impairment of their phagocytic ability and an increase in pro-inflammatory gene expression [42]. These results indicate the presence of a multi-directional intercellular communication network in ALS that is mediated by miRNAs encapsulated in EVs. Researchers have only begun to scratch the surface of EV-mediated miRNA transfer in ALS and this area requires more comprehensive study to fully disentangle the pathologic milieu that exists among the different types of nerve cells in ALS nervous tissue.

Research investigating EV-mediated ALS pathophysiology is in an incipient stage, and impressive results in previous studies are still raising a number of important questions that must be addressed. For example, it is unclear whether the beneficial effect of elimination of intracellular toxic proteins outweighs the deleterious effects of uptake of those proteins by neighboring cells. Understanding this point will be critical when designing therapeutic methods to inhibit the propagation process. Furthermore, to promote extracellular disposal of toxic protein aggregates while inhibiting their uptake by neighboring cells, we need to fully understand the interactions between surface proteins on detrimental EVs and those on the plasma membranes of motor neurons. Alternatively, efforts could be focused on enhancing lysosomal degradation process over EV-mediated protein disposal in diseased cells, but it is unclear whether the majority of detrimental contents in their multivesicular bodies can alternatively be delivered to autophagosomes for degradation. Another gap in EV-ALS research is a lack of studies focused on analyzing motor neuron-derived EVs to understand the phenotypic effect of transmitting neuron-originated proteins to other neurons and/or non-neuronal cells within ALS tissues. As motor neurons are the main target in ALS pathogenesis, pathogenic proteins are likely to be enriched in motor neuron-derived EVs and could potentially directly damage glia and/or NMJ structures, or even directly affect skeletal muscle contractility. We believe that answering these questions, in addition to better characterizing non-neuronal EV cargos, should constitute the principle focuses of future studies aimed at improving our understanding of EV-mediated ALS progression. The results of such work would doubtlessly provide invaluable insights into ALS pathophysiology and help identify suitable targets for future therapeutic development.

3. Can EVs serve as reliable biomarkers for ALS?

There is no reliable biomarker established for ALS, neither for confirming disease onset nor for characterizing disease progression [43]. The lack of a reliable biomarker for ALS makes the correct prognosis challenging, and even limits diagnosis to relatively late stages, after patients recognize their neuromuscular symptoms. As the typical life expectancy for ALS patients is approximately 2–5 years after disease onset, early and accurate diagnosis is crucial not only for developing early-stage applicable therapies, but for improving quality of life for patients during their follow-up period. A new detection method should be robust and convenient for clinical settings, and, critically, have sufficient detection sensitivity, specificity, and reproducibility to ensure confidence in the result. Meeting all these requirements simultaneously is an extremely challenging goal, given the extremely heterogeneous nature of the disease. Recent studies are evaluating ALS patient-derived EVs as potential biomarkers of ALS for prognosis, early diagnosis, and patient stratification. RNAs collected from patient's blood or cerebrospinal fluid (CSF;

often used as a surrogate for nervous tissue sampling) are the main target of analyses so far and advanced RNA-sequencing techniques are being employed to analyze deregulated RNAs exclusively in ALS patient-derived EVs. Recently, Otake et al. reported a new methodology using highly sensitive exoRNA-sequencing for comprehensive analysis of exosomal mRNAs in patient CSF, to identify abnormally expressed mRNAs in exosome samples from ALS patients [43]. The technique identified 543 mRNAs exhibiting statistically different expression patterns compared to normal samples. In particular, this analysis revealed that the gene *CUEDC2* was only detected in ALS patient-derived exosomes. As the gene is known to regulate the ubiquitin-proteasome pathway as part of the inflammatory response, its abnormal expression is postulated to cause potential neuroinflammation in ALS, making *CUEDC2* mRNA a strong biomarker candidate [43]. Follow-up studies are necessary to demonstrate a specific causal relationship between exosomal *CUEDC2* mRNA presence (rather than free intracellular *CUEDC2* expression) and ALS development. Furthermore, work demonstrating an omnipresence of the same RNA mis-regulation in EVs from other ALS patients is also required. However, the described study highlights how exosomal mRNAs could be attractive biomarker candidates, given their stability within body fluids, as well as the convenience of sample collection and ease of subsequent data analysis. Efforts to date to characterize EV cargos as ALS biomarkers, including those discussed in detail above and below, are summarized in **Table 2**.

As non-coding RNAs are also reported to be involved in ALS onset and progression, miRNAs loaded in EVs represent another candidate biomarker class for ALS diagnosis. Study of free miRNA for ALS detection has been previously reported. Microarray analyses were performed on ALS mutant mouse-derived cells and patient serum, and the results identified the expression of 10–13 dysregulated miRNAs in diseased samples [44, 45]. In addition to free-miRNA analyses, Saucier et al. tried identifying ALS-associated miRNA signatures in EVs to discriminate blood between healthy and ALS individuals. Extensive exosomal RNA analysis using high-throughput sequencing coupled with droplet digital PCR enabled the identification of a group of dysregulated miRNAs, including miR-183-5p, miR-9-5p, miR-338-3p and miR-1246, which were all remarkably downregulated in ALS patient-derived exosomes [45].

EV-based biomarker studies in ALS have so far given promising results and strong motivation for follow-up studies to further specify molecular candidates with higher disease relevancy. However, limited information on the exosomal RNAs, in terms of the specific signaling pathways they regulate, is currently available. This lack of understanding makes it difficult to determine the relevance of each when attempting to define a diagnostic EV-RNA signature for ALS. Also, as significant difficulty lies in identifying the cellular origin of EVs collected from body fluids, their practical application in diagnostics could be challenging, especially if the same miRNAs secreted from different cells of origin reflect different states of the disease. Furthermore, the RNA profile in different subtypes of EVs, such as exosomes versus microvesicles, that exist in patient's body fluids has not yet been investigated. As such, more comprehensive RNA analysis, using entire EV populations, might give discordant results to those reported from exosomal RNA analysis. Additionally, to date there has not been any analysis of when specific RNAs arise during ALS disease progression and whether certain expression patterns are indicative of certain stages of the pathology. Such an understanding is crucial in determining whether expression of certain RNAs can be employed effectively as diagnostic tools or as methods to chart disease progression. Finally, as hundreds of exosomal RNAs in ALS patient body fluids have been found to exhibit significant differences in their expression levels relative to normal controls, clinically

Role of EV	Study method	Source of EV	Significance	Unknowns	Reference
Biomarker	Sequencing exosomal mRNAs in CSF	CSF of ALS patients and normal donors	A new methodology for comprehensive analysis of exosomal mRNAs in human CSF using newly developed exoRNA-seq, which showed potential applicability to identify specific ALS biomarkers	Specificity level of mRNAs detected in ALS exosome using the technique	Otake et al. [43]
	Clinical study comparing the expression of miR-27a-3p in serum-derived exosomes	Serum of ALS patients and healthy subjects	The expression of miR-27a-3p in patients with ALS was significantly downregulated than that in healthy human serum exosomes	Specific role of miR-27-3p in the expression of disease phenotypes in ALS	Xu et al. [63]
	Clinical analysis of miRNA profile in 16 ALS patients	Serum of ALS patients and healthy controls	Distinct miRNA expression profile was observed in ALS patient's serum-derived exosomes compared to healthy controls	Are ALS-associated miRNAs actually involved in post-transcriptional regulation of neurons?	Saucier et al. [45]
	In vitro study with NSC-34 and N9 microglia to discover ALS specific miRNAs	Motor neuron like NSC-34 cells with mSOD1 expression	Increased level of miR-124 in circulating exosomes of NSC-34 may be used as potential biomarker of motor neuron degeneration in ALS	miR-124 expression in other health state? (false positive issue)	Pinto et al. [42]
Therapeutic agent	*In vitro* study using adipose-derived stem cells and human SOD1 overexpressing mouse NSCs	Adipose-derived stem cells	Adipose-derived stem cell exosomes showed paracrine effect to SVG neurons to alleviate their disease phenotypes and mitochondrial dysfunction in ALS	Major exosomal cargos that exert each of therapeutic effects on recipient neurons	Lee et al. [48]
	In vitro study assessing efficacy of stromal cell-derived exosomes on NSC-34 cells expressing hSOD1 mutants	Murine adipose-derived stromal cells	The ASC-derived exosomes were able to protect motor neuron-like NSC-34 (SOD1 mutant) from oxidative stress and increase their viability	Where does the beneficial effect of ASC-exosomes come from?	Bonafede et al. [50]
	Proteomic profiling of exosomes derived from mASC	Murine adipose-	Proteomic analysis revealed mASC-derived exosomes	Exosomal effect on actual restoration of	Bonafede et al. [47]

Role of EV	Study method	Source of EV	Significance	Unknowns	Reference
	with *in vitro* assay of exosome treatment on NSC-34 cells	derived stem cells	contain proteins for cell adhesion and negatively regulate cell apoptosis	neuronal function	

Table 2.
Summary of the applications of extracellular vesicles in ALS diagnosis and treatment.

applicable diagnosis will be difficult until we better understand the physiological outcomes of those misregulated RNAs in neuromuscular tissue maintenance and function. Future research elucidating the expression patterns of EV cargos across diverse ALS populations at different disease stages, as well as studies of the signaling pathways regulated by EV-RNAs in ALS tissue, are therefore necessary before the value of these molecules in ALS diagnostic medicine can be fully evaluated.

4. EVs for therapeutic agents in ALS treatment

EVs hold distinct advantages for function as stable biomolecule carriers. Their lipid bilayers, decorated with transmembrane proteins, protect cargo molecules from enzymatic degradation in the extracellular space as well as making them immune-tolerant. Functional transmembrane proteins also promote EV internalization into recipient cells, which naturally occurs through active fusion of EV membranes with cell's plasma membranes. This in turn facilitates release of EV molecular cargo to recipient cell cytoplasms or induces endosome uptake for functional activation [23, 46].

Accordingly, an attractive hypothesis is that therapeutic molecules loaded in vesicles could be delivered to target cells to subsequently modulate phenotypes in neurodegenerative disease. In such a model, cargo molecules could encompass proteins and mRNAs, or non-coding RNAs for post-transcriptional protein regulation, or even specific compounds for sustained activation with avoidance of enzymatic attack. Research efforts to test this hypothesis are summarized in **Table 2** and discussed in detail below. As very few drug candidates with a proven efficacy for treating ALS exist, research on 'drug-loaded EVs' has not yet begun in earnest. However, adipose-derived stromal cells and stem cells have shown a capacity to generate exosomes capable of conferring a therapeutic effect on defective neurons. Exosomes from murine adipose-derived stromal cells alleviated oxidative stress and reduced hydrogen peroxide-induced apoptosis in NSC-34 cells overexpressing a human SOD1 mutant variant [47]. Safe availability and a capacity to migrate to damaged tissues for their reparative processes make stromal cells good candidates for EV sources. Although the study demonstrated that stromal cell-derived EVs can reverse SOD-1 induced cell death, such applications have not yet been specifically targeted to restore electrophysiological phenotypes in ALS neurons. Consequentially, the applicability of stromal cell-derived EVs may be limited if the specific cargo molecule responsible for restoring motor neuron function is not identified.

Retaining the remarkable therapeutic potential of stem cells, while avoiding issues with tumorigenicity, insufficient therapeutic specificity, and substantial cell loss during treatment, stem cell-derived EVs offer an exciting alternative to direct stem cell therapy. Indeed, EVs obtained from undifferentiated stem cells have shown a capacity to alleviate disease phenotypes in ALS mutant neurons. Specifically, exosomes from adipose-derived stem cells reduced SOD1 aggregation and

DOI: http://dx.doi.org/10.5772/intechopen.91388

rescued normal mitochondrial protein expression in mouse neurons [48]. Another adipose-derived stem cell study performed proteomic analysis of EVs and found 189 exosomal proteins, mainly involved in regulating cell adhesion and negative regulation of apoptosis. Stress response proteins, such as SOD1, were also included in these exosomes and were found to replace the enzymatic function of mutant SOD1 in NSC-34 cells. Additionally, the study reported the presence of ribonuclease RNase 4 in the examined exosomes. This could represent a potential neuroprotective molecule applicable in ALS, as RNase 4 has been reported to have angiogenic, neuroprotective properties [49, 50].

The field of EV-mediated therapeutics for ALS treatment is still in its infancy. However, since glial cells and neural stem cells are responsible for regulating neuron differentiation, protection, and synaptic function [13, 51–54], EVs derived from those cells could constitute attractive subcomponents for therapeutic agent development. As mentioned above, EVs possess distinct advantages for therapeutic development, including sustained cargo delivery and avoidance of physiological degradation. Naturally derived EVs, as well as engineered EVs loaded with optimal therapeutic materials, therefore represent a powerful candidate for the future of ALS treatment. However, the following issues should be addressed to facilitate the practical application of EVs in treating this disease. First, since EVs secreted from one type of cell usually do not target a specific cell type for cargo delivery, higher delivery specificity to eliminate potential off-target effects is essential. EV membrane engineering to attach proteins with exclusive affinity to target neuron cell surfaces could be an attractive approach to consider [55–58], if reliable surface markers for diseased cells can be defined. Second, a lack of information regarding the physiological function of specific cargo molecules in glia or stem cell-derived EV limits their applicability in ALS treatment. As disease phenotypes in ALS are extremely heterogeneous, investigating the role of each EV-loadable molecule with more categorized efficacy studies beyond cell viability is also highly required. Production scale of EVs is a critical issue for the actual application of this technology in ALS clinics. Although EV collection technology continues to advance to minimize EV loss and reduce collection time and cost, most EV experiments are still done in small-scale benchtop studies. This is not a huge issue during these early stages of research and development, but will cause a critical problem for scale up and

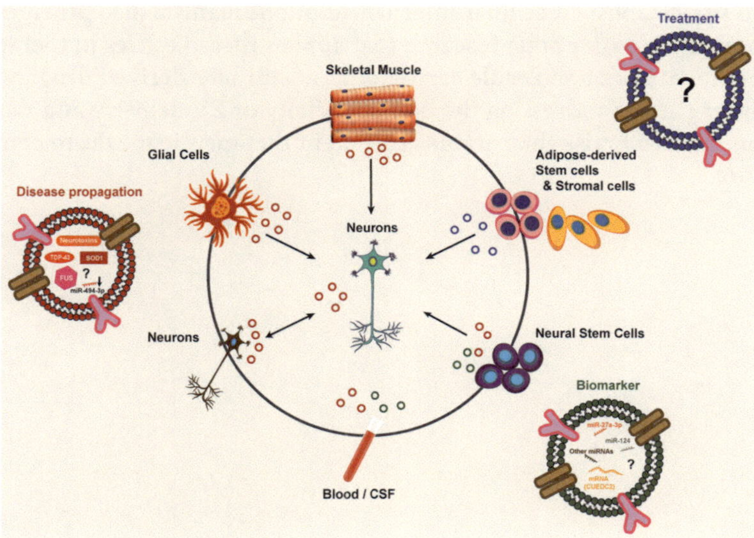

Figure 1.
Schematic summary of the major role EVs play in ALS propagation, diagnosis, and treatment.

administration as we move closer to clinical trials and subsequent distribution. Lastly, cargo molecule purity is another significant issue. Even with a single cell source, EV cargo composition is likely to be different based on culture conditions, and may fluctuate due to other unknown factors; especially if cell-derived EVs is advanced to large-scale production (**Figure 1**).

5. Conclusions

Current EV research in relation to ALS is weighted toward investigating the pathogenic role of intercellularly transmissible vesicles, with a particular focus on dysregulated protein propagation. This is likely due to the fact that SOD1 and TDP-43 mutant cells are already known to produce neurotoxic protein aggregates, which makes the hypothesis that their dissemination via EVs contributes to the nature of irreversible degeneration of neuromuscular tissue in ALS a straightforward one. Several studies have demonstrated that EVs collected from ALS patient's body fluids and from mutant non-neuronal cells can be internalized by healthy cells. Their capacity to induce neurodegenerative behavior in these cells supports the notion that these structures contribute to the rapid disease progression characteristic of ALS. However, the effect of collected EV components in specific ALS disease phenotypes is currently quite ambiguous, especially for correlating neuromuscular tissue level abnormalities with defined EV component expression. To address this, EV-mediated interplay, occurring at the diseased NMJ may be a good potential target for future investigations. EVs secreted from skeletal muscle and motor neurons are known to contribute significantly to the development of normal synaptic formation at the NMJ and better understanding how these signaling processes are disrupted in ALS could significantly improve our understanding of early disease etiology. Work in these early stages of ALS and EVs has also highlighted the potential for using EVs as either a biomarker for ALS diagnostics or even a potential therapeutic agent. Although evidence of a causal relationship between misregulated EV-RNAs and functional impairments in ALS neurons is currently sparse, notable differences in ALS EV-RNA expression patterns detected by next generation sequencing does support their potential as future diagnostic tool. EV's exogenous nature and pre-established cellular internalization mechanism also provides substantial motivation to continue research that applies these vesicles in therapy development, either as a molecule carrier or as a naturally-derived drug in and of itself. Further studies addressing the non-specificity of EV delivery and issues with production scale will raise their status as a potent therapeutic means to combat ALS in the future.

Author details

Changho Chun[1], Alec S.T. Smith[1,2,4], Mark Bothwell[2,4] and David L. Mack[1,3,4]*

1 Department of Bioengineering, The University of Washington, Seattle, WA, United States

2 Department of Physiology and Biophysics, The University of Washington, Seattle, WA, United States

3 Department of Rehabilitation Medicine, The University of Washington, Seattle, WA, United States

4 The Institute for Stem Cell and Regenerative Medicine, Seattle, WA, United States

*Address all correspondence to: dmack21@uw.edu

References

[1] Valko K, Ciesla L. Amyotrophic lateral sclerosis. Progress in Medicinal Chemistry. 2019;**58**:63-117

[2] Pansarasa O et al. Sod1 in amyotrophic lateral sclerosis: "Ambivalent" behavior connected to the disease. International Journal of Molecular Sciences. 2018;**19**:1-13

[3] Niedermeyer S, Murn M, Choi PJ. Respiratory failure in amyotrophic lateral sclerosis. Chest. 2019;**155**: 401-408

[4] Ferrara D, Pasetto L, Bonetto V, Basso M. Role of extracellular vesicles in amyotrophic lateral sclerosis. Frontiers in Neuroscience. 2018;**12**:1-9

[5] Roy J, Saucier D, O'Connell C, Morin P. Extracellular vesicles and their diagnostic potential in amyotrophic lateral sclerosis. Clinica Chimica Acta. 2019;**497**:27-34

[6] Scotter EL, Chen H, Shaw CE. TDP-43 proteinopathy and ALS: Insights into disease mechanisms and therapeutic targets. Neurotherapeutics. 2015;**12**: 352-363

[7] Silverman JM et al. CNS-derived extracellular vesicles from superoxide dismutase 1 (SOD1) G93A ALS mice originate from astrocytes and neurons and carry misfolded SOD1. The Journal of Biological Chemistry. 2019;**294**: 3744-3759

[8] Barmada SJ et al. Autophagy induction enhances TDP43 turnover and survival in neuronal ALS models. Nature Chemical Biology. 2014;**10**: 677-685

[9] Paolicelli RC, Bergamini G, Rajendran L. Cell-to-cell communication by extracellular vesicles: Focus on microglia. Neuroscience. 2019; **405**:148-157

[10] Pascua-Maestro R et al. Extracellular vesicles secreted by astroglial cells transport apolipoprotein D to neurons and mediate neuronal survival upon oxidative stress. Frontiers in Cellular Neuroscience. 2019;**12**:1-13

[11] Lee Y, El Andaloussi S, Wood MJA. Exosomes and microvesicles: Extracellular vesicles for genetic information transfer and gene therapy. Human Molecular Genetics. 2012;**21**: 125-134

[12] Hessvik NP, Llorente A. Current knowledge on exosome biogenesis and release. Cellular and Molecular Life Sciences. 2018;**75**:193-208

[13] Frühbeis C, Fröhlich D, Krämer-Albers EM. Emerging roles of exosomes in neuron-glia communication. Frontiers in Physiology. 2012;**3**:1-7

[14] Basso M, Bonetto V. Extracellular vesicles and a novel form of communication in the brain. Frontiers in Neuroscience. 2016;**10**:1-13

[15] Pegtel DM, Gould SJ. Exosomes. Annual Review of Biochemistry. 2019; **88**:487-514

[16] Pluta R, Ułamek-Kozioł M, Januszewski S, Czuczwar SJ. Exosomes as possible spread factor and potential biomarkers in Alzheimer's disease: Current concepts. Biomarkers in Medicine. 2018;**12**:1025-1033

[17] Vingtdeux V et al. Alkalizing drugs induce accumulation of amyloid precursor protein by-products in luminal vesicles of multivesicular bodies. The Journal of Biological Chemistry. 2007;**282**:18197-18205

[18] Jan AT et al. Perspective insights of exosomes in neurodegenerative diseases: A critical appraisal. Frontiers in Aging Neuroscience. 2017;**9**:1-8

[19] Sardar Sinha M et al. Alzheimer's disease pathology propagation by exosomes containing toxic amyloid-beta oligomers. Acta Neuropathologica. 2018;**136**:41-56

[20] Rajendran L et al. Alzheimer's disease β-amyloid peptides are released in association with exosomes. Proceedings of the National Academy of Sciences of the United States of America. 2006;**103**:11172-11177

[21] Janas AM, Sapoń K, Janas T, Stowell MHB, Janas T. Exosomes and other extracellular vesicles in neural cells and neurodegenerative diseases. Biochimica et Biophysica Acta, Biomembranes. 2016;**1858**:1139-1151

[22] Mulcahy LA, Pink RC, Raul D, Carter F. Routes and mechanisms of extracellular vesicle uptake. Journal of Extracellular Vesicles. 2014;**1**:1-14

[23] Saeedi S, Israel S, Nagy C, Turecki G. The emerging role of exosomes in mental disorders. Translational Psychiatry. 2019;**9**:122

[24] Wainger BJ et al. Intrinsic membrane hyperexcitability of ALS patient-derived motor neurons. Cell Reports. 2014;**7**:1-11

[25] Ramesh N, Pandey UB. Autophagy dysregulation in ALS: When protein aggregates get out of hand. Frontiers in Molecular Neuroscience. 2017;**10**:1-18

[26] Basso M et al. Mutant copper-zinc superoxide dismutase (SOD1) induces protein secretion pathway alterations and exosome release in astrocytes: Implications for disease spreading and motor neuron pathology in amyotrophic lateral sclerosis. The Journal of Biological Chemistry. 2013;**288**: 15699-15711

[27] Berning BA, Walker AK. The pathobiology of TDP-43 C-terminal fragments in ALS and FTLD. Frontiers in Neuroscience. 2019;**13**:1-27

[28] Xu ZS. Does a loss of TDP-43 function cause neurodegeneration? Molecular Neurodegeneration. 2012;**7**:1

[29] Solomon DA et al. A feedback loop between dipeptide-repeat protein, TDP-43 and karyopherin-α mediates C9orf72-related neurodegeneration. Brain. 2018;**141**:2908-2924

[30] Smethurst P et al. In vitro prion-like behaviour of TDP-43 in ALS. Neurobiology of Disease. 2016;**96**:236-247

[31] Mitra J et al. Motor neuron disease-associated loss of nuclear TDP-43 is linked to DNA double-strand break repair defects. Proceedings of the National Academy of Sciences of the United States of America. 2019;**116**: 4696-4705

[32] Bilican B et al. Mutant induced pluripotent stem cell lines recapitulate aspects of TDP-43 proteinopathies and reveal cell-specific vulnerability. Proceedings of the National Academy of Sciences. 2012;**109**:5803-5808

[33] Zondler et al. Impaired activation of ALS monocytes by exosomes. Immunology & Cell Biology. 2017;**95**: 207-214

[34] Grad LI, Pokrishevsky E, Silverman JM, Cashman NR. Exosome-dependent and independent mechanisms are involved in prion-like transmission of propagated Cu/Zn superoxide dismutase misfolding. Prion. 2014;**8**: 331-335

[35] Rashed MH et al. Exosomes: From garbage bins to promising therapeutic targets. International Journal of Molecular Sciences. 2017;**18**:538

[36] Iguchi Y et al. Exosome secretion is a key pathway for clearance of pathological TDP-43. Brain. 2016;**139**: 3187-3201

[37] Feiler MS et al. TDP-43 is intercellularly transmitted across axon terminals. The Journal of Cell Biology. 2015;**211**:897-911

[38] Nonaka T et al. Prion-like properties of pathological TDP-43 aggregates from diseased brains. Cell Reports. 2013;**4**: 124-134

[39] Turner MR, Goldacre R, Ramagopalan S, Talbot K, Goldacre MJ. Autoimmune disease preceding amyotrophic lateral sclerosis: An epidemiologic study. Neurology. 2013; **81**:1222-1225

[40] Pagani MR, Gonzalez LE, Uchitel OD. Autoimmunity in amyotrophic lateral sclerosis: Past and present. Neurology Research International. **2011**; **2011**:497080

[41] Varcianna A et al. Micro-RNAs secreted through astrocyte-derived extracellular vesicles cause neuronal network degeneration in C9orf72 ALS. eBioMedicine. 2019;**40**:626-635

[42] Pinto S, Cunha C, Barbosa M, Vaz AR, Brites D. Exosomes from NSC-34 cells transfected with hSOD1-G93A are enriched in mir-124 and drive alterations in microglia phenotype. Frontiers in Neuroscience. 2017;**11**:273

[43] Otake K, Kamiguchi H, Hirozane Y. Identification of biomarkers for amyotrophic lateral sclerosis by comprehensive analysis of exosomal mRNAs in human cerebrospinal fluid. BMC Medical Genomics. 2019;**12**:1-11

[44] Waller R et al. Small RNA sequencing of sporadic amyotrophic lateral sclerosis cerebrospinal fluid reveals differentially expressed miRNAs related to neural and glial activity. Frontiers in Neuroscience. 2018;**11**:1-13

[45] Saucier D et al. Identification of a circulating miRNA signature in extracellular vesicles collected from amyotrophic lateral sclerosis patients. Brain Research. 2019;**1708**:100-108

[46] Guitart K et al. Improvement of neuronal cell survival by astrocyte-derived exosomes under hypoxic and ischemic conditions depends on prion protein. Glia. 2016;**64**:896-910

[47] Bonafede et al. The anti-apoptotic effect of ASC-exosomes in an in vitro ALS model and their proteomic analysis. Cells. 2019;**8**:1087

[48] Lee M et al. Adipose-derived stem cell exosomes alleviate pathology of amyotrophic lateral sclerosis in vitro. Biochemical and Biophysical Research Communications. 2016;**479**:434-439

[49] Li S et al. NIH Public Access. 2014; **16**:387-404

[50] Bonafede R et al. Exosome derived from murine adipose-derived stromal cells: Neuroprotective effect on in vitro model of amyotrophic lateral sclerosis. Experimental Cell Research. 2016;**340**: 150-158

[51] Dzyubenko E, Gottschling C, Faissner A. Neuron-glia interactions in neural plasticity: Contributions of neural extracellular matrix and perineuronal nets. Neural Plasticity. **2016;2016**:5214961

[52] Farhy-Tselnicker I, Allen NJ. Astrocytes, neurons, synapses: A tripartite view on cortical circuit development. Neural Development. 2018;**13**:1-12

[53] Bellot-Saez A, Kékesi O, Morley JW, Buskila Y. Astrocytic modulation of neuronal excitability through K+spatial buffering. Neuroscience and Biobehavioral Reviews. 2017;**77**:87-97

[54] Rakic P, Lombroso PJ. Development of the cerebral cortex: I. Forming the cortical structure. Journal of the

American Academy of Child and Adolescent Psychiatry. 1998;**37**:116-117

[55] Cheng H et al. Chimeric peptide engineered exosomes for dual-stage light guided plasma membrane and nucleus targeted photodynamic therapy. Biomaterials. 2019;**211**:14-24

[56] Vogt S, Stadlmayr G, Grillari J, Rüker F, Wozniak-Knopp G. Engineering of surface proteins in extracellular vesicles for tissue-specific targeting. Current Topics in Biochemical Engineering. 2019:1-21. DOI: 10.5772/intechopen.83537

[57] Antes TJ et al. Targeting extracellular vesicles to injured tissue using membrane cloaking and surface display. Journal of Nanobiotechnology. 2018;**16**:1-15

[58] Yang Y, Hong Y, Cho E, Kim GB, Kim IS. Extracellular vesicles as a platform for membrane-associated therapeutic protein delivery. Journal of Extracellular Vesicles. 2018;**7**:1440131

[59] Sproviero D et al. Pathological proteins are transported by extracellular vesicles of sporadic amyotrophic lateral sclerosis patients. Frontiers in Neuroscience. 2018;**12**:1-9

[60] Gall et al. Secretion of toxic exosomes by muscle cells of ALS patients: Role in ALS pathogenesis. Neuromuscular Disorders. 2017;**27**:S32

[61] Westergard T et al. Cell-to-cell transmission of dipeptide repeat proteins linked to C9orf72-ALS/FTD. Cell Reports. 2016;**17**:645-652

[62] Zhou et al. Exosomes released by human umbilical cord mesenchymal stem cells protect against cisplatin-induced renal oxidative stress and apoptosis in vivo and in vitro. Stem Cell Research & Therapy. 2013;**4**:34

[63] Xu Q et al. Comparison of the extraction and determination of serum exosome and miRNA in serum and the detection of miR-27a-3p in serum exosome of ALS patients. Intractable & Rare Diseases Research. 2018;**7**:13-18

Chapter 6

The Extraocular Muscles Are Selectively Spared in ALS

Fatima Pedrosa Domellöf

Abstract

The extraocular muscles differ from other skeletal muscles in many respects but most strikingly in their response to neuromuscular diseases expected to affect the whole body. Oculomotor disturbances are not typical features of ALS. Recent data ascribe the muscle tissue an important role in the pathophysiology of ALS, with early involvement of the neuromuscular junctions and loss of axonal contact. We show that the extraocular muscles of terminal ALS donors and also of mice models of ALS maintain their morphology and well-preserved neuromuscular junctions until the end stages of the disease, whereas the limb muscles are severely affected and their neuromuscular junctions start losing contact with the supplying axons early in the course of ALS. There are intrinsic differences between the extraocular and limb muscles with respect to neurotrophic factors and Wnt isoforms and fundamental differences in their response to ALS that cannot be explained by the aging process. We propose that these differences may be instrumental in the selective sparing of the extraocular muscles in ALS.

Keywords: extraocular muscle, ALS, pathophysiology, neurotrophic factor, neuromuscular junction, Wnt, BDNF, GDNF, NT-3, NT-4, S-100B, synaptophysin, p75, neurofilament, Wnt1, Wnt3a, Wnt5a, Wnt7

1. Introduction

Amyotrophic lateral sclerosis (ALS) is a late-onset progressive neurodegenerative disorder affecting both the upper and lower motor neurons. It is characterized by increasing muscle weakness, paresis, and paralysis, and although the course of the disease may vary considerably, death usually occurs within 3–5 years due to respiratory failure. While almost all skeletal muscles, including the cranially innervated muscles responsible for speech and swallowing, are affected in ALS, oculomotor disturbances are not dominant or typical features of this disease, not even in patients with long-duration ALS, and eye movements may remain the only form of communication available to these patients at the end stages of the disease. The cranial nerve nuclei supplying the eye muscles appear rather normal in terminal ALS patients [1], and abnormalities in eye motility in ALS patients, when present, have been ascribed to supranuclear deficits [2].

The pathophysiology of the neurodegenerative process in ALS has been proposed to be due to a number of different causes. The traditional point of view has been that ALS is a motor neuron disease that progresses to the periphery where it affects the muscles, due to the typical loss of motor neurons in the anterior horns of the spinal cord and sclerosis of the lateral corticospinal tracts. However, a number of studies suggest an inverse course of events, with changes starting at the periphery and progressing along the motor neurons toward the CNS, reviewed by [3–5]. In SOD1G93A transgenic mice, it has been shown that peripheral denervation occurs in the limb muscles before the animals become clinically weak or motor neuron loss is detected [6]. Similar results were also reported for a patient with ALS who died unexpectedly, leading the authors to propose that motor neuron pathology in ALS begins at the distal axon end and proceeds in a "dying back" pattern [6]. Later, it has been shown that muscle-restricted expression of three different SOD1 gene variants can initiate the non-autonomous degeneration of motor neurons typical of ALS [7], truly showing that the muscle itself may be a major player in the early stages of ALS.

A unifying model compiling extensive experimental data from SOD1 transgenic models of ALS [3] proposes that although motor neuron degeneration and death are the primary causes of the progressive paralysis, neighboring nonneuronal cells are also involved in the toxicity and damage development. In this model, the earliest event is the retraction of motor axons from their muscle synapses, before any symptoms of the disease are present.

The extraocular muscles (EOMs) are unique in many respects and are considered a separate muscle class, allotype. They are both the fastest and the most fatigue-resistant muscles in the body, and their fiber-type composition is very complex [8, 9]. The unique properties of the EOMs are reflected in their expression profile that differs from that of limb muscle in over 300 genes [10]. However, the most striking property of EOMs is their varied behavior in disease. The EOMs are known to be selectively involved in certain diseases like mitochondrial myopathies, myasthenia gravis, and Miller Fisher syndrome, but preferentially spared in other devastating diseases like Duchenne muscular dystrophy and merosin-deficient muscular dystrophy, that affect all other muscles in the body [11–13].

The extraocular muscles are richly innervated, and their motor units are very small, with 7–25 muscle fibers, in contrast to the motor units of limb muscles, which typically contain hundreds of muscle fibers. The majority of the nerve fibers in the EOMs are large and myelinated and innervate a typical single "en plaque" endplate in the middle portion of each muscle fiber. The remaining 15–20% of the EOM nerve fibers are small and innervate many small, "en grappe" motor endplates along the length of a muscle fiber (the so-called multiply innervated muscle fibers, reviewed in [11]). This traditional description of the innervation of the EOMs has been significantly changed by the recent report of a subpopulation of muscle fibers that exhibit multiple large "en plaque" nerve endings [14]. The NMJs of the EOMs also differ from limb muscle in retaining expression of the fetal gamma subunit of the acetylcholine receptor (AChR), in addition to the adult epsilon subunit, typically present in mature motor endplates [14, 15]. We have shown that the NMJs of the human EOMs have a different immunoreactivity pattern than that seen in limb muscles for antibodies against gangliosides GQ1b, GT1a, and GD1b [16]. Gangliosides are a large family of sialylated glycosphingolipids highly enriched in neuronal and glial plasma membranes and important for the development, function, and maintenance of the nervous system. Complex gangliosides have neurotrophic factor-like activity and may regulate the expression levels of neurotrophic factors and their receptors [17]. Notably, there have been at least two case reports of ALS associated with antibodies against gangliosides [18, 19].

Given that the EOMs differ significantly from the limb and trunk muscles with respect to their response to disease and given the more recent view that the muscle itself may play a key role in the pathophysiology of ALS, we first investigated whether there are any major differences between the EOMs and the limb muscles of terminal ALS donors [20]. Thereafter, we investigated neuromuscular junction integrity [21–23], neurotrophic factors (BDNF, NT-3, NT-4, GDNF) and their receptors (p75NTR, TrkB, TrkC) [24, 25], and relevant Wnt isoforms (Wnt1, Wnt3a, Wnt5a, Wnt7a) [26], as possible important puzzle pieces to better understand the pathophysiology of ALS and the selective sparing of the EOMs in the disease.

2. The extraocular muscles of terminal ALS donors are remarkably well preserved

We compared the general morphology, fiber-type content, fiber area and myosin heavy chain (MyHC) composition of EOM, biceps brachii, vastus lateralis, and tibialis anterior muscle samples collected from eight terminal ALS donors (age 58–80 years) and from three age-matched (age 72–86 years) and a younger (age 26 years) control, with ethical approval, using immunohistochemistry and SDS-PAGE [20]. There were five cases of sporadic ALS and three cases of familial ALS. The MyHC isoforms are the major determinants of key contractile and biochemical characteristics of the myofibers including shortening velocity and power and therefore very good markers of the physiological properties of myofibers. Our study showed that the morphology of the ALS limb muscle samples is clearly pathological. All limb muscle samples from terminal ALS donors exhibit typical signs of myofiber type grouping, myofiber splitting, necrosis, increased connective tissue, fatty replacement, and ongoing regeneration, with a very wide range of myofiber areas. In contrast, the EOM samples from the same donors show remarkably well-preserved morphology. In 18 out of the 43 EOM samples examined, larger variation in fiber area was apparent than in the control samples and irrespectively of being sporadic or familial ALS cases. In fact, areas that appear well preserved reveal a general atrophy of all myofiber types, whereas areas that appear more affected generally show atrophy of the myofibers containing MyHCslow and hypertrophy of the myofibers containing MyHCfast2A. In 20 EOM samples, increased connective tissue amounts were noted, either around individual myofibers or around groups of myofibers. The changes noticed vary among donors and among different EOM samples from a given donor. Centrally placed nuclei are rarely detected. The MyHC content, determined with SDS-PAGE of whole EOM extracts, varies among ALS donors, whereas it is rather similar among control EOM samples [20]. This variation in MyHC content at the whole muscle level can be interpreted as reflecting different levels of involvement, and, to a lesser degree, naturally occurring variation among subjects [8].

Given that this first study clearly shows that the human EOMs are remarkably well preserved at the end stage of ALS [20] and because the EOMs are known to show a divergent behavior in disease, we decided to further investigate these muscles in ALS, comparing the EOMs and limb muscle samples from human donors and from mouse models of ALS, taking a "muscle perspective" to study the pathophysiology of the disease.

3. Maintained neuromuscular junction occupancy in the extraocular muscles at end stages of ALS

In the SOD1G93A mouse, the most widely used mouse model of ALS, it has been shown that loss of contact between the axons and the myofibers, at the neuromuscular junctions, occurs early in the course of the disease and indeed precedes detection of loss of motor neurons in the spinal cord [6]. Similar findings have been reported in ALS patients who died of other reasons early in the course of ALS [6]. Furthermore, data show that muscle-specific alterations are sufficient to trigger neuromuscular pathology and distal degeneration of motor neurons [5, 7], suggesting that the muscle itself may play an important role in the pathophysiology of ALS.

We investigated [21] whether there are signs of loss of contact between the axons and the myofibers, at the neuromuscular junctions of the EOMs, extensor digitorum longus, tibialis anterior, and gastrocnemius and soleus muscles from seven SOD1G93A transgenic and six control mice. We used triple labeling immunohistochemistry with antibodies against neurofilament protein and synaptophysin to identify the axonal side of the neuromuscular junctions and their axons and alpha-bungarotoxin, to identify the muscle side of the neuromuscular junctions, in the same muscle section. Our study confirmed that, as described above for the human EOMs of terminal ALS donors, the eye muscles in this animal model of ALS also show rather well-preserved morphological features, in clear contrast to the limb muscles of the same animal, at the end stage of the disease. We could confirm previously reported findings [6] of significant loss of contact between the nerve and myofiber in approximately 33% of the neuromuscular junctions in limb muscles of the ALS mouse model, whereas in the limb muscles of the control animals, only approximately 4.6% of the neuromuscular junctions lack contact with the supplying nerve ($p = 0.0071$). In contrast, the number of neuromuscular junctions lacking nerve contacts in the EOMs is extremely low and similar between transgenic (1.9%) and control (1.7%) animals ($p = 0.659$) [21].

Similarly, the neuromuscular junctions of the EOMs of terminal ALS donors show maintenance of their integrity [22, 23]. In a study of 7 terminal ALS donors (age 58–80 years, three cases with SOD1D90A genotype) and 10 controls (adults aged 34–53 years and elderly aged 69–83 years), we compared the EOMs and the limb muscles with respect to the presence and distribution of neurofilament light subunit (marker of the axons in nerves and at the neuromuscular junction), synaptophysin (marker of synaptic vesicles and thereby of functioning neuromuscular junctions), S100B, $p75^{NTR}$ and glial fibrillary acidic protein (GFAP) which are markers of terminal Schwann cells at the neuromuscular junction, and alpha-bungarotoxin, which labels the muscle side of the synapse [23]. GFAP and $p75^{NTR}$ are upregulated in Schwann cells after injury [27–29]. Two groups of control donors (adult and elderly) were included in this and all our studies of ALS in order to distinguish between the effects of normal aging and those related to ALS. This pioneer study showed that there is a dramatic decrease in the number of neuromuscular junctions and nerve axons containing neurofilament light subunit in limb muscles of terminal ALS donors, whereas the EOMs maintain neurofilament light subunit in their neuromuscular junctions and nerves. There is also a significant decrease in neuromuscular junctions labeled with synaptophysin in the limb muscles but not in the EOMs of terminal ALS donors. Together, these results confirm that there is a marked loss of nerve-muscle contacts in the limb muscles of terminal ALS donors, whereas the EOMs succeed in maintaining their neuromuscular junctions until the end stage of the disease. The neuromuscular junctions of limb muscles show also massive loss of S100B and $p75^{NTR}$ in ALS, whereas the staining pattern of GAFP is maintained. In contrast, the neuromuscular junctions in the EOMs of terminal ALS donors also show loss of S100B but have an unchanged pattern regarding the other two Schwann cell markers, GFAP and $p75^{NTR}$. The loss of S100B can be interpreted as due to downregulation rather than a sign of loss of Schwann cells, given that the other two markers remain unchanged. It may also indicate a disturbed calcium homeostasis as an early step toward the loss of the neuromuscular junction in ALS. In summary, this study shows fundamental differences between the limb muscles and the EOMs of terminal ALS donors with a significant impact of the disease on important synaptic proteins normally present in the motor axons and terminal Schwann cells in the limb muscles, whereas the neuromuscular junctions in the EOMs are only very mildly affected [23].

Another study has in addition revealed fragmentation of the postsynaptic membrane, decreased density of acetylcholine receptors, and absence of nerve sprouting in denervated neuromuscular junctions in the limb muscles of the SOD1G93A mouse model of ALS, whereas no such changes are present in the neuromuscular junctions of the EOMs of the same animals [30].

In the context of motor axon retraction from the muscle synapse being an early event in the pathogenesis of ALS, it is of particular interest to further investigate the cellular and molecular microenvironment of the neuromuscular junctions of the extraocular muscles, as they may provide cues to the unique resistance of the EOMs to ALS.

4. Important differences in neurotrophic factors between extraocular and limb muscles

Alterations in the expression of target-derived neurotrophic factors and in their signaling pathways have been reported in ALS. Neurotrophic factors are important for survival and maintenance of neurons [31–33]. Target-derived neurotrophic factors can be transported to lower motor neurons from other cells, including the muscle cells, by retrograde transport, and from upper motor neurons, by anterograde transport, and act as signaling molecules [31–33]. Among neurotrophic factors, brain-derived neurotrophic factor (BDNF) is of particular interest due to its capacity to promote motor neuron survival and motor axon growth [32–34]. Glial cell line-derived neurotrophic factor (GDNF) is also relevant as it is capable of rescuing motor neurons from injury-induced cell death [35], and neurothrophin-4 (NT-4) plays a role in growth and remodulation of adult motor neurons [36, 37], whereas NT-3 is of particular importance for sensory neurons.

Data on the SOD1G93A mouse model of ALS show important differences between the EOMs and the limb muscles over time regarding the levels of expression of neurotrophic factors [24]. The authors compared the expression levels of BDNF, GDNF, NT-3, and NT-4, determined with quantitative RT-PCR, in limb (soleus and gastrocnemius) and extraocular muscles at the early stage (50 days) and at the end stage (150 days) of the disease. Starting with the control animals, the EOMs differ from the limb muscles by having significantly lower levels of BDNF and NT-3 mRNA at age 50 days. At 150 days, the control EOMs have significantly lower levels of BDNF and NT-4 mRNA than the limb muscles from the same animals. In the limb muscles of control animals, mRNA levels of BDNF increase significantly from 50 to 150 days of age, whereas the levels of NT-3 decrease dramatically. In the control EOMs, the mRNA levels of BDNF, GDNF, NT-3, and NT-4 remain unchanged from 50 to 150 days of age [24].

In the transgenic animals, the expression levels of BDNF increase significantly from 50 to 150 days, that is, from the early stage of ALS, when the limb muscle morphology is still normal, to the end stage of the disease, when the limb muscles are extremely affected. Compared to the controls, the limb muscles of the transgenic animals show significantly lower levels of NT-4 at 50 days and significantly higher levels of GDNF at 150 days. The transgenic EOMs show no change in the levels of expression of BDNF or GDNF and show significant decrease in NT-3 and increase in NT-4, over time between 50 and 150 days, and the morphology is comparable to that of the age-matched controls. Compared to the controls, the EOMs of the G93A animals show significantly higher levels of GDNF and NT-3 at 50 days, whereas no significant differences are detectable at 150 days. Finally, comparison between the EOMs and limb muscles of transgenic animals shows no significant differences in the levels of expression of any of the four neurotrophic factors at 50 days but significantly higher levels of BDNF in the limb muscles at 150 days [24].

Because no significant changes in the levels of expression of BDNF detected with quantitative RT-PCR are apparent in either the limb or EOMs of the transgenic animals at any stage, the authors dismiss a possible role for this neurotrophic factors on ALS. The BDNF results obtained in the SOD1G93A mice are in agreement with a previous report from muscle samples of ALS patients [38]. In contrast, the GDNF mRNA levels are significantly upregulated in the EOMs of the SOD1G93A mice at 50 days, and the authors suggest that this early upregulation is triggered by the disease and seminal for the maintenance of the general morphology of the EOMs and in particular for their capacity of keeping intact neuromuscular junctions. They interpret the upregulation of GDNF in the end stage in the limb muscles as reflecting the advanced motor neuron degeneration. Similarly, the upregulation of NT-3 in the EOMs detected at 50 days is also proposed to be triggered by ALS and to protect the EOMs, whereas early downregulation of NT-4 in the limb muscles is suggested to be detrimental and contribute to the loss of axonal contact at the neuromuscular junctions [24].

At the cellular level, there are also important differences in the patterns of distribution of neurotrophic factors between the EOMs and limb muscles, both among controls and among SOD1G93A animals at 50 and 150 days [25]. In the limb muscles of control animals, GDNF, BDNF, NT-3, and NT-4 are present in the vast majority of the neuromuscular junctions at 50 and 150 days, whereas that is the case in only a little over half of the neuromuscular junctions in the control EOMs, at 50 and 150 days. The proportion of neuromuscular junctions containing BDNF and NT-4 is significantly higher in the limb muscles than in the EOMs of control animals at 50 days, and the same is true for the proportion of neuromuscular junctions containing BDNF and GDNF at 150 days. Particularly noteworthy is that the limb muscles of SOD1G93A animals show a significant decrease in the proportion of neuromuscular junctions containing BDNF, GDNF, and NT-4 at 150 days, whereas the EOMs maintain their pattern. The same is true for the presence of the receptors $p75^{NTR}$, TrkB, and TrkC, which decline significantly in the neuromuscular junctions of the limb muscles of the SOD1G93A animals at 150 days, but not in their EOMs. TrkB is a high-affinity tyrosine kinase receptor specific for BDNF and NT-4, TrkC is a high-affinity tyrosine kinase receptor specific for NT-3, and $p75^{NTR}$ is a low-affinity receptor for BDNF, NT-3, and NT-4 [39]. There are only discrete differences between the control and the SOD1G93A animals with respect to patterns of neurotrophic factors in the nerve axons and the myofibers of both EOM and limb muscles [25].

Taken together, these studies [24, 25] clearly show both at the mRNA level and immunohistochemically that the EOMs have lower neurotrophic factor levels than the limb muscles, in control mice. One possible explanation resides in the differences in innervation between these muscles, as the EOMs have a rich population of multiply innervated myofibers, in contrast to the exclusively twitch myofibers of limb muscles, and the developmental fates of these different types of axons are dependent upon target-derived neurotrophic factors [40]. They also show that the significant changes in neurotrophic factors in limb muscles of transgenic animals are not related to normal aging.

Studies of neurotrophic factors in muscle tissue pose a technical challenge and clinical trials in ALS have not led to the desired effects, but the early detection of alterations in the levels of expression of neurotrophic factors and the distinct patterns observed in the EOMs versus limb muscles indicate that it is too early to dismiss their possible roles in the pathophysiology of ALS and in particular in the selective capacity of the EOMs to maintain neuromuscular junctions and remain rather unaffected in the disease.

5. Differences in Wnt profiles between extraocular and limb muscles

Several Wnt proteins, including Wnt1, Wnt3a, Wnt 5a, and Wnt7a, are highly expressed at the neuromuscular junction, in muscle fibers, and in motor neurons, and abnormal Wnt signaling has been reported in ALS and a number of other neuromuscular conditions [41–46]. In particular, Wnt1 has been assigned important roles in muscle regeneration and in synaptic plasticity, acting on both sides of the synapse [41, 47]. Wnt3a modulates the formation of neuromuscular junctions and promotes nerve outgrowth [48–50], whereas Wnt5a is important for motor neuron survival during development [51]. Wnt7a plays an important role in synaptic assembly and plasticity and remodeling of incoming axons [52] and has also been shown to have positive effects on the myofibers [53, 54]. Furthermore, Riluzole, the only medical treatment available for ALS, enhances Wnt/beta catenin signaling.

We have performed a comprehensive immunohistochemical study comparing the distribution of Wnt1, Wnt3a, Wnt5a, and Wnt7a in the EOMs and limb muscle samples (biceps brachii, vastus lateralis, and tibialis anterior) from six terminal ALS donors, younger controls (mean age 41 years for EOMs and 33 years for limb muscles, referred to as adult controls), and older controls (mean age 75 years for EOM and 76 years for limb, referred to as elderly controls), and we have reported significant differences and suggested a role for Wnts in the different behaviors of EOMs and limb muscles in ALS [26].

In the adult control EOMs, roughly 71% of the axons are Wnt1 positive, and in the elderly controls, merely 12% of the axons contain Wnt1, whereas in the EOMs of terminal ALS donors, 43% of axons are labeled for Wnt1, clearly showing that they preferentially maintain Wnt1 in their nerves. The limb muscles of terminal ALS donors contain significantly less Wnt1-positive axons than the EOMs, with extremely high variation among the different donors. No statistically significant differences between the three limb muscle groups are detectable regarding the presence of Wnt1 in the motor nerves. Wnt1 is present in almost 40% of the myofibers in the EOMs of adult controls and almost in all myofibers of terminal ALS donors, whereas it is not present in limb myofibers of adult controls or terminal ALS donors.

With regard to Wnt3a, it is present in the vast majority of axons in both the EOMs of adult controls and ALS terminal donors, but again it is significantly lower in the elderly control EOMs. In the limb muscles of all groups, the percentage of axons containing Wnt3a is significantly lower than in the EOMs, with approximately 75% fewer Wnt3a axons. Approximately 17% of the myofibers contain Wnt3a in adult control EOM, whereas almost all myofibers in the EOMs of terminal ALS donors are positive. Higher levels of Wnt3a are present in adult control limb myofibers, but in contrast Wnt3a is practically absent in the limb muscle fibers of terminal ALS donors.

Wnt5a is present in practically all EOM axons both in adult controls and terminal ALS donors and is somewhat lower in the EOMs of elderly controls. Similarly, practically all limb muscle axons, irrespective of group, are Wnt5a positive. Wnt5a, seen as weak immunostaining, is present in almost all myofibers of control adult EOMs and terminal ALS donors, whereas it is not present in limb myofibers of adult controls or terminal ALS donors.

A very large proportion of the axons in the EOMs of adult controls and terminal ALS donors are Wnt7a positive, whereas a significantly lower number is found in the EOMs of the elderly controls. A similar proportion of Wnt7a-positive axons are present in the limb muscles of both adult controls and terminal ALS donors, but a significantly higher number of positive axons are found in the limb muscles of elderly controls. Only approximately 20% of the myofibers in the adult control EOMs contain Wnt7a, but in the EOMs of terminal ALS donors, this number increases significantly almost 60%. In the limb muscles, Wnt7a is present in more than half of the myofibers of the adult controls and practically in all myofibers in the elderly controls. The differences found between adult controls and terminal ALS donors regarding Wnt7a in limb myofibers are not significant, probably due to large interindividual variation among the donors.

Data collected in controls and in the SOD1G93A mouse model of ALS [26] indicates that practically all neuromuscular junctions in control EOMs and limb muscles express Wnt1, Wnt3a, Wnt5a, and Wnt7 at 50 and 150 days. The same is true for the transgenic EOMs at both 50 and 150 days and the transgenic limb muscles at 50 days, whereas a significantly decrease in the proportion of neuromuscular junctions co-expressing the different Wnt isoforms is clearly apparent in the transgenic limb samples at 150 days.

6. Summary

In summary, the EOMs remain remarkably well preserved until the end stages of ALS, both in human terminal donors and in mouse models of ALS. They maintain the composition of their neuromuscular junctions and do not loose contact with the supplying axon. Furthermore, important differences exist between the EOMs and the limb muscles with respect to neurotrophic factors and Wnts:

- The mRNA levels of BDNF, NT-4, and NT-3 and the detection of BDNF, NT-4, NT-3, and GDNF at the protein level are lower in the EOMs than in the limb muscles of control animals at 50 and/or 150 days.

- NT-3 is upregulated in the EOMs of SOD1G93A mice at 50 days and may be protective. A similar difference in GDNF may also be advantageous for the EOMs and protect their motor neurons.

- There is early downregulation of NT-4 in the limb muscles of SOD1G93A mice compared to the controls at the same age, which coincides with the timing of early loss of motor axon occupancy at the neuromuscular junctions of limb muscles in this ALS model [6].

- The proportion of neuromuscular junctions in the EOMs positive for BDNF, GDNF, and NT-4 is not changed between the controls and the transgenic mice at 150 days, whereas there is a significant decrease in the limb muscles of the SOD1G93A animals compared to the controls at late stage and there is also a significant decrease over the course of the disease in the limb muscles of the transgenic mice. Again, these changes in neurotrophic factors parallel the loss of axonal occupancy at the neuromuscular junctions of the limb muscles of transgenic animals and these neurotrophic factors are known to play crucial roles in regulating the synapses [55, 56].

- There is a significant decrease in the neurotrophic factor receptors p75NTR, TrkB, TrkC, and GFR-alpha1 in the neuromuscular junctions of terminal SOD1G93A mice, whereas they are maintained in the neuromuscular junctions of terminal transgenic EOMs.

- Wnt1 and Wnt3a are present in a larger proportion of axons in the human control EOMs than in the limb muscles. The myofibers in the control EOMs contain higher Wnt1 and Wnt5a and lower Wnt3a and Wnt7a than the myofibers of limb muscles, and although the exact implications of these intrinsic differences in Wnt isoform profiles remain to be determined, they may be relevant for the selective sparing of the EOMs in ALS.

- Wnt1 and Wnt3a are present at significantly higher levels in the axons and the muscle fibers of the EOMs than in the axons or muscle fibers of the limb muscles of terminal ALS donors. Because Wnt1 plays a role in synaptic plasticity and muscle regeneration and in neuromuscular junction formation during fetal development and Wnt3a has similar roles, these differences between EOMs and limb muscles are likely to be of importance for the selective sparing of the EOMs, and in particular of their neuromuscular junctions, in ALS.

Altogether, these data show important differences between the EOMs and limb muscles with regard to neurotrophic factors and four different Wnt isoforms, both at base line and in ALS, that likely play a role in the selective sparing of the EOMs in ALS. These data also suggest that muscle itself may provide a door for the development of new treatment strategies in the future.

Conflict of interest

There are no conflicts of interest.

Author details

Fatima Pedrosa Domellöf
Department of Clinical Science, Ophthalmology, Umeå University, Umeå, Sweden

*Address all correspondence to: fatima.pedrosa-domellof@umu.se

References

[1] Sobue G, Matsuoka Y, Mukai E, Takayanagi T, Sobue I, Hashizume Y. Spinal and cranial nerve roots in amyotrophic lateral sclerosis and X-linked recessive bulbospinal muscular atrophy: Morphometric and teased-fiber study. Acta Neuropathologica. 1981;**55**:227-235

[2] Donaughy C, Thurtell MJ, Pioro EP, Gibson JM, Leigh RJ. Eye movements in amyotrophic lateral sclerosis and its mimics: A review with illustrative cases. Journal of Neurology, Neurosurgery, and Psychiatry. 2011;**82**:110-116

[3] Boillée S, Vande Velde C, Cleveland DW. ALS: A disease of motor neurons and their nonneuronal neighbors. Neuron. 2006;**52**:39-59

[4] Loeffler JP, Picchiarelli G, Dupuis L, Gonzalez De Aguilar JL. The role of skeletal muscle in amyotrophic lateral sclerosis. Brain Pathology. 2016;**26**(2):227-236

[5] Dupuis L, Loeffler J-P. Neuromuscular junction destruction during amyotrophic lateral sclerosis: Insights from transgenic models. Current Opinion in Pharmacology. 2009;**9**:341-346

[6] Fischer RL, Culver DG, Tennant P, et al. Amyotrophic lateral sclerosis is a distal neuropathy: Evidence in mice and man. Experimental Neurology. 2004;**185**:232-240

[7] Wong M, Martin L. Skeletal muscle-restricted expression of human SOD1 causes motor neuron degeneration in transgenic mice. Human Molecular Genetics. 2010;**19**:2284-2302

[8] Kjellgren D, Thornell L-E, Pedrosa-Domellöf F. Myosin heavy chain isoforms in human extraocular muscles. Investigative Ophthalmology & Visual Science. 2003;**44**:1419-1425

[9] Kjellgren D, Ryan M, Ohlendieck K, Thornell L-E, Pedrosa-Domellöf F. Sarco(endo) plasmic reticulum Ca2+ ATPases (SERCA 1 and 2) in human extraocular muscles. Investigative Ophthalmology & Visual Science. 2003;**44**:5057-5062

[10] Fischer MD, Gorospe JR, Felder E, Bogdanovich S, Pedrosa-Domellöf F, Ahima RS, et al. Expression profiling reveals metabolic and structural components of extraocular muscle. Physiological Genomics. 2002;**9**:71-84

[11] Sadeh M. Extraocular muscles. In: Engel AG, Franzini-Armstrong C, editors. Myology. New York: McGraw-Hill; 2004. pp. 119-127

[12] Pedrosa-Domellöf F. Extraocular muscles: Extraocular muscle involvement in disease. In: Dartt DA, Besharse JC, Dana R, editors. Encyclopedia of the Eye. Vol. 2. Oxford: Academic Press; 2010. pp. 99-104

[13] Pedrosa-Domellöf F. Extraocular muscles: Response to neuromuscular diseases and specific pathologies. In: McLoon LM, Andrade FH, editors. Craniofacial Muscles: A New Framework for Understanding the Effector Side of Craniofacial Muscle Control. New York: Springer; 2012. pp. 75-90

[14] Liu J-X, Pedrosa Domellöf F. A novel type of multiterminal motor endplate in human extraocular muscles. Investigative Ophthalmology & Visual Science. 2018;**59**:539-548

[15] Kaminski HJ, Kusner LL, Block CH. Expression of acetylcholine receptor isoforms in extraocular muscle endplates. Investigative Ophthalmology & Visual Science. 1996;**37**:345-351

[16] Liu J-X, Willison HJ, Pedrosa-Domellöf F. Immunolocalisation of

GQ1b and related gangliosides in human extraocular neuromuscular junctions and muscle spindles. Investigative Ophthalmology & Visual Science. 2009;**50**:3226-3232

[17] Kittaka D, Itoh M, Ohmi Y, et al. Impaired hypoglossal nerve regeneration in mutant mice lacking complex gangliosides: Down-regulation of neurotrophic factors and receptors as possible mechanisms. Glycobiology. 2008;**18**:509-516

[18] Mizutani K, Oka N, Kusunoki S, et al. Amyotrophic lateral sclerosis with IgM antibody against gangliosides GM2 and GD2. Internal Medicine. 2003;**42**:277-280

[19] Yamazaki T, Suzuki M, Watanabe T, et al. Amyotrophic lateral sclerosis with IgG anti-GalNAc-GD1a antibodies. Clinical Neurology and Neurosurgery. 2008;**110**:722-724

[20] Ahmadi M, Liu J-X, Brännström T, Andersen PM, Stål P, Pedrosa-Domellöf F. Human extraocular muscles in amyotrophic lateral sclerosis. Investigative Ophthalmology & Visual Science. 2010;**51**:3494-3501

[21] Tjust A, Brännström T, Pedrosa DF. Unaffected motor endplate occupancy in extraocular muscles of ALS G93A mouse model. Frontiers in Bioscience. 2012;**4**:1547-1555

[22] Liu J-X, Brännström T, Andersen PM, Pedrosa-Domellöf F. Different impact of ALS on laminin isoforms in human extraocular muscles versus limb muscles. Investigative Ophthalmology & Visual Science. 2011;**52**:4842-4852

[23] Liu J-X, Brännström T, Andersen PM, Pedrosa Domellöf F. Distinct changes in synaptic protein composition at neuromuscular junctions of extraocular muscles versus limb muscles of ALS donors. PLoS One. 2013;**8**(2):e57473

[24] Harandi VM, Lindquist S, Kolan SS, Brannström T, Liu JX. Analysis of neurotrophic factors in limb and extraocular muscles of mouse model of amyotrophic lateral sclerosis. PLoS One. 2014;**9**(10):e109833

[25] Harandi VM, Gaied ANR, Brännström T, Pedrosa Domellöf F, Liu J-X. Unchanged neurotrophic factors and their receptors correlate with sparing in extraocular muscles in amyotrophic lateral sclerosis. Investigative Ophthalmology & Visual Science. 2016;**57**:6831-6842

[26] McLoon LK, Harandi VM, Brännström T, Andersen PM, Liu J-X. Wnt and extraocular muscle sparing in amyotrophic lateral sclerosis. Investigative Ophthalmology & Visual Science. 2014;**59**:322-329

[27] Triolo D, Dina G, Lorenzetti I, Malaguti M, Morana P, et al. Loss of glial fibrillary acidic protein (GFAP) impairs Schwann cell proliferation and delays nerve regeneration after damage. Journal of Cell Science. 2006;**119** (Pt 19):3981-3993

[28] Bussmann KA, Sofroniew MV. Re-expression of p75NTR by adult motor neurons after axotomy is triggered by retrograde transport of a positive signal from axons regrowing through damaged or denervated peripheral nerve tissue. Neuroscience. 1999;**91**(1):273-281

[29] Scott AL, Ramer MS. Schwann cell p75NTR prevents spontaneous sensory reinnervation of the adult spinal cord. Brain. 2010;**133**(Pt 2):421-432

[30] Valdez G, Tapia JC, Lichtman JW, Fox MA, Sanes JR. Shared resistance to aging and ALS in neuromuscular junctions of specific muscles. PLoS One. 2012;**7**:e34640

[31] Pitts EV, Potluri S, Hess DM, Balice-Gordon RJ. Neurotrophin and Trk-mediated signaling in the neuromuscular system. International Anesthesiology Clinics. 2006;**44**(2):21-76

[32] Henderson CE, Camu W, Mettling C, Gouin A, Poulsen K, Karihaloo M, et al. Neurotrophins promote motor neuron survival and are present in embryonic limb bud. Nature. 1993;**363**(6426):266-270

[33] Sendtner M, Holtmann B, Kolbeck R, Thoenen H, Barde YA. Brain-derived neurotrophic factor prevents the death of motoneurons in newborn rats after nerve section. Nature. 1992;**360**(6406):757-759

[34] Yan Q, Elliott J, Snider WD. Brain-derived neurotrophic factor rescues spinal motor neurons from axotomy-induced cell death. Nature. 1992;**360**(6406):753-755

[35] Henderson CE, Phillips HS, Pollock RA, Davies AM, Lemeulle C, Armanini M, et al. GDNF: A potent survival factor for motoneurons present in peripheral nerve and muscle. Science. 1994;**266**(5187):1062-1064

[36] Funakoshi H, Belluardo N, Arenas E, Yamamoto Y, Casabona A, Persson H, et al. Muscle-derived neurotrophin-4 as an activity-dependent trophic signal for adult motor neurons. Science. 1995;**268**(5216):1495-1499

[37] Beaumont E, Gardiner PF. Endurance training alters the biophysical properties of hindlimb motoneurons in rats. Muscle & Nerve. 2003;**27**(2):228-236

[38] Grundström E, Lindholm D, Johansson A, Blennow K, Askmark H. GDNF but not BDNF is increased in cerebrospinal fluid in amyotrophic lateral sclerosis. Neuroreport. 2000;**11**(8):1781-1783

[39] Chao MV, Hempstead BL. p75 and Trk: A two-receptor system. Trends in Neurosciences. 1995;**18**(7):321-326

[40] Oppenheim RW, Prevette D, Haverkamp LJ, Houenou L, Yin QW, McManaman J. Biological studies of a putative avian muscle-derived neurotrophic factor that prevents naturally occurring motoneuron death in vivo. Journal of Neurobiology. 1993;**24**(8):1065-1079

[41] Ataman B, Ashley J, Gorczyca M, Ramachandran P, Fouquet W, Sigrist SJ, et al. Rapid activity-dependent modifications in synaptic structure and function require bidirectional Wnt signaling. Neuron. 2008;**57**(5):705-718

[42] Cisternas P, Henriquez JP, Brandan E, Inestrosa NC. Wnt signaling in skeletal muscle dynamics: Myogenesis, neuromuscular synapse and fibrosis. Molecular Neurobiology. 2014;**49**(1):574-589

[43] Packard M, Koo ES, Gorczyca M, Sharpe J, Cumberledge S, Budnik V. The drosophila Wnt, wingless, provides an essential signal for pre- and postsynaptic differentiation. Cell. 2002;**111**(3):319-330

[44] Korkut C, Budnik V. WNTs tune up the neuromuscular junction. Nature Reviews Neuroscience. 2009;**10**(9):627-634

[45] Tury A, Tolentino K, Zou Y. Altered expression of atypical PKC and Ryk in the spinal cord of a mouse model of amyotrophic lateral sclerosis. Developmental Neurobiology. 2014;**74**(8):839-850

[46] Yu L, Guan Y, Wu X, Chen Y, Liu Z, Du H, et al. Wnt signaling is altered by spinal cord neuronal dysfunction in amyotrophic lateral sclerosis transgenic mice. Neurochemical Research. 2013;**38**(9):1904-1913

[47] Salinas PC, Zou Y. Wnt signaling in neural circuit assembly. Annual Review of Neuroscience. 2008;**31**:339-358

[48] Endo T. Molecular mechanisms of skeletal muscle development, regeneration, and osteogenic conversion. Bone. 2015;**80**:2-13

[49] David MD, Canti C, Herreros J. Wnt-3a and Wnt-3 differently stimulate proliferation and neurogenesis of spinal neural precursors and promote neurite outgrowth by canonical signaling. Journal of Neuroscience Research. 2010;**88**(14):3011-3023

[50] Henriquez JP, Webb A, Bence M, Bildsoe H, Sahores M, Hughes SM, et al. Wnt signaling promotes AChR aggregation at the neuromuscular synapse in collaboration with agrin. Proceedings of the National Academy of Sciences of the United States of America. 2008;**105**(48):18812-18817

[51] Agalliu D, Takada S, Agalliu I, McMahon AP, Jessell TM. Motor neurons with axial muscle projections specified by Wnt4/5 signaling. Neuron. 2009;**61**(5):708-720

[52] Salinas PC. Retrograde signaling at the synapse: A role for Wnt proteins. Biochemical Society Transactions. 2005;**33**:1295-1298

[53] von Maltzahn J, Bentzinger CF, Rudnicki MA. Wnt7a-Fzd7 signalling directly activates the Akt/mTOR anabolic growth pathway in skeletal muscle. Nature Cell Biology. 2011;**14**(2):186-191

[54] von Maltzahn J, Renaud JM, Parise G, Rudnicki MA. Wnt7a treatment ameliorates muscular dystrophy. Proceedings of the National Academy of Sciences of the United States of America. 2012;**109**(50):20614-20619

[55] Je HS, Yang F, Ji Y, Potluri S, Fu XQ, Luo ZG, et al. ProBDNF and mature BDNF as punishment and reward signals for synapse elimination at mouse neuromuscular junctions. The Journal of Neuroscience. 2013;**33**(24):9957-9962

[56] Lu B, Nagappan G, Guan X, Nathan PJ, Wren P. BDNF-based synaptic repair as a disease-modifying strategy for neurodegenerative diseases. Nature Reviews Neuroscience. 2013;**14**(6):401-416

Section 3

Novel Therapeutics and Challenges

Chapter 7

RNA Metabolism and Therapeutics in Amyotrophic Lateral Sclerosis

Orietta Pansarasa, Stella Gagliardi, Daisy Sproviero and Cristina Cereda

Abstract

Amyotrophic lateral sclerosis (ALS) is a progressive neuromuscular disorder characterized by the selective death of upper and lowers motor neurons in spinal cord, brain stem, and motor cortex, which leads to paralysis and death within 2–3 years of onset. Deeply sequencing technologies, to simultaneously analyze the transcriptional expression of thousands of genes, offered new possibilities to focus on ALS pathogenesis and, most notably, to find new potential targets for novel treatments. The present book chapter illustrates recent advances in transcriptomic studies in animal models and human samples and in new molecular targets related to ALS pathogenesis and disease progression. Additionally, new insights into the involvement of altered transcriptional profiles of noncoding RNAs (microRNA and lncRNA) and ALS-associated ribosomal binding proteins have been investigated, to understand the functional consequences of extensive RNA dysregulation in ALS. Attention has been also turned on how transcriptome alterations could highlight new molecular targets for drug development.

Keywords: ALS, RNA metabolism, transcriptomics, gene expression, noncoding RNA

1. Introduction

Highlights

- Aberrant RNA metabolism is one of the major contributors to ALS pathogenesis.
- Understanding RNA-binding protein functions and identifying target RNA regulatory networks is crucial to deepen ALS knowledge and to develop new therapeutics.
- miRNAs are strongly linked to the development of ALS and are indicated as new potential biomarkers.
- lncRNAs have been recently indicated to play important roles in CNS in health and disease such as ALS.
- miRNA-based therapeutics as well as deregulated AS are considered important areas for therapeutic intervention.

Amyotrophic lateral sclerosis (ALS) is a progressive and fatal neurodegenerative disorder (ND) that affects the human motor system, that is, the lower and upper motor neurons (MNs). Among the symptoms of ALS, there are progressive muscle weakness and paralysis, swallowing difficulties, and breathing impairment due to respiratory muscle weakness that finally causes death, within 2–5 years following clinical diagnosis [1]. Now, also extramotor systems are involved in ALS, thus providing new insight into the pathogenesis of the disease. So far, no effective therapy is available for ALS: Rilutek (riluzole) and Radicava (edaravone) are the only two drugs approved by the Food and Drug Administration for ALS treatment. Unfortunately their effect in slowing disease progression is very modest [2]. The majority of ALS cases, named as sporadic (sALS), has no a family history; a fraction of cases (about 5–10%) are considered familial (fALS) [3], because of mutations in genes involved in a wide range of cellular functions. 60–70% of fALS and 10% of sporadic ALS (sALS) cases can be ascribed to mutations in SOD1, TARDBP, FUS, VCP, C9ORF72, and OPTN [4]; further rare genetic variants have also been identified, MATR3, HNRNPA1, HNRNPA2/B1, EWSR1, TAF15, ANG, UBQLN2, VAPB, TBK1, SQSTM1, PFN1, TUBA4A, KIF5A, ANXA11, and CHCHD10 [5]. Although an in-depth understanding of the mechanisms underlying ALS has yet to be reached, a growing interest was addressed to the impairment of RNA metabolism as one of the major contributor to ALS pathogenesis. This concept is reinforced by the discovery of genetic mutations in FUS and in TARDBP genes coding for RNA binding proteins (RBPs), which play a multifaceted role in transcription and in maintaining RNA metabolism. Recent studies have reported that a substantial portion of the genome is actively transcribed as noncoding RNA molecules. These noncoding RNAs are fundamental key actors in the regulation of biological processes and function as a "fine switch" of gene expression. It is now recognized that dysregulations in the noncoding RNAs gene expression is a putative mechanism in several neurological disorders, including ALS. Moreover, noncoding RNAs are emerging as new potential biomarkers contributing to an early disease diagnosis and treatment follow-up. To date, miRNA have been one the main focus of most ALS studies. miRNAs are differentially expressed in several tissues (CSF, plasma and serum) in ALS patients compared to healthy controls.

In this chapter, we will focus on the involvement of altered transcriptional profiles of microRNAs (miRNAs) and long noncoding RNA (lncRNA) as well as on ALS-related RNA binding proteins. We also review biomarkers and potential therapeutic strategies based on the manipulation of noncoding RNAs.

2. Dysfunctions in RNA metabolism and RNA-binding protein

It is broadly recognized that an aberrant RNA metabolism may contribute to RNA toxicity, which is due to the accumulation of toxic RNAs and to the dysfunction of RBPs [6].

Messenger RNAs (mRNAs) are subjected to several processing steps including splicing, polyadenylation, editing, transport, translation, and turnover. All these processes are extremely dynamic and require the involvement of RBPs to coordinate both co- and posttranscriptional processing of transcripts. Understanding RBPs functions and identifying their target RNA regulatory networks are crucial to deepen the knowledge in NDs and to promptly develop new therapeutics.

Nussbacher and colleagues by a genome-wide approach, have shed a new light on how RBPs may affect the fate of their targets [7]. Considering the great impact of RBPs on the expression, splicing, and translation of multiple RNA targets, also little changes in their expression and/or activity have amplified effects. Moreover, an altered interaction between RBPs and their targets can induce serious pathological phenotypes, even if the exact mechanism is not clear. Briefly, we focus on RBPs,

TARDBP and FUS, and SOD1 and C9orf72 to highlight recent progresses on their involvement in RNA dysregulation.

TDP-43 is a heterogeneous nuclear RBP of 414 amino acids that contains two RNA recognition motifs (RRM1-2), a glycine rich domain in the C-terminus and nuclear localization and export signals (NLS and NES) [8, 9]. TDP-43 is crucial in RNA processing, that is, RNA splicing, transcription, transport, stability, as well as miRNA production [10]. TDP-43 binds to more than 6000 RNA targets in the brain [11, 12]. TDP-43 binds to mRNA and regulates the expression of other proteins: FUS, Tau, ATXN2 CHMP2B, VAPB, and progranulin, all involved in ALS and in other NDs [12, 13]. Polymenidou and colleagues using an RNA-seq approach, demonstrated the involvement of TDP-43 in the regulation of the expression of 239 mRNAs, many of those encoding synaptic proteins including neurexin NRXN1-3, neuroligin NLGN1-2, Homer2, microtubule-associated protein 1B (MAP1B), GABA receptors subunits (GABRA2, GABRA3), AMPA receptor subunits (GRIA3, GRIA4), syntaxin 1B, and calcium channels [11, 14–17]. Together these data suggest the involvement of TDP-43 in neuronal morphology, synaptic transmission, and neuronal plasticity likely through the regulation of RNA processing of synaptic genes [14]. TDP-43 is also a splicing regulator which decreases its own expression level by binding to the 3′-untranslated (UTR) region of its own pre-mRNA [18]. Moreover, its depletion or overexpression can influence the alternative splicing of specific targets genes, which are altered in ALS [11, 13, 19]. In 2012, Kawahara and Mieda-Sato also demonstrated the involvement of TDP-43 in miRNA biogenesis. TDP-43 helps the production of the precursor miRNAs (pre-miRNAs) through the interaction of the Drosha complex and the binding to the primary miRNAs (pri-miRNAs) [20]. An increased expression of miR-633 and a decreased expression of the let-7b miRNA have been observed when TDP-43 is downregulated [21]. Moreover, TDP-43 binds to lncRNAs, including the nuclear-enriched autosomal transcript 1 (NEAT1) and metastasis-associated lung adenocarcinoma transcript 1 (MALAT1) [13]. Until now, the exact role of this interaction is unclear; however both NEAT1 and MALAT1 levels are enhanced in patients with frontotemporal lobar degeneration (FTLD) and ALS [12, 22]. Nishimoto and co-authors identified paraspeckles, that is, membraneless nuclear bodies, with high levels of NEAT1 and TDP-43 in MNs of patients in the early stage of the disease [22], thus interfering with TDP-43-mediated RNA processing and disrupting RNA homeostasis in ALS MNs.

FUS is an RBP of 526 amino acids mainly located in the nuclei. It is composed by an RNA recognition motif, a SYGQ (serine, tyrosine, glycine, and glutamine)-rich region, several RGG (arginine, glycine, and glycine)-repeat regions, a C2C2 zinc finger motif, and a nuclear localization signal (NLS) [23]. Similar to TDP-43, FUS has a key role in RNA processing. It is involved in transcriptional regulation, mRNA splicing, and miRNA production. FUS co-modulates certain transcription factors, including NF-kB, SPI1, and Runbox transcription factor (RUNX) [24, 25]. Genome-wide approaches have evidenced more than 5000 human RNA targets for FUS [26]. Considering that FUS is part of the hnRNP complex, it is crucial for the splicing mechanism [23], and it may affect the splicing mechanism of more than 900 mRNAs [26]. Among these, FUS may regulate the alternative splicing of genes related to cytoskeletal organization, axonal growth, and guidance such as the microtubule-associated protein tau (MAPT) [27], Netrin G1 (NTNG1) [28], neuronal cell adhesion molecule (NRCAM), and the actin-binding LIM (ABLIM1) [29]. Like TDP-43, FUS also binds to different mRNAs of ALS-related genes, VCP, VAPB, ubiquilin-2, and OPTN, thus modulating their expression [12, 26]. Furthermore, FUS is involved in the biogenesis of miRNA by recruiting Drosha to pri-miRNAs at their transcription sites and supports the biogenesis of a subset of miRNAs [30]. However, if FUS directly regulates the function of mature miRNAs remains to be understand. Finally, FUS is crucial for the regulation of NEAT 1 levels and paraspeckle formation. FUS nuclear deficiency, its loss of nuclear function, as well as its aggregation might cause sequestration of paraspeckle components into pathological inclusions. Thus, the interaction between FUS and NEAT 1 is involved in the development of neuronal dysfunction in ALS [31].

SOD1 is not an RBP; however, several authors demonstrated that mutant SOD1 has a role in RNA metabolism regulation [32, 33]. These authors reported that mutant SOD1 can bind mRNA species, that is, vascular endothelial growth factor (VEGF) and neurofilament light chain (NFL), and alter their expression, stabilization, and function [32, 33]. Mutant SOD1, by the direct bind to the 3' UTR of VEGF mRNA, promotes the sequestration of other RBPs such as TIA-1-related protein (TIAR) and Hu antigen R (HuR) into insoluble aggregates. This, in turn, determines the impairment of HuR function and interferes with the HuR neuroprotective effect during stress responses [32]. Chen and colleagues further demonstrated that, through the modification of neurofilament (NF) stoichiometry, mutant SOD1 destabilizes NFL mRNA. Consequently, NFs aggregate in MNs and are considered a hallmark of ALS disease [33]. NFL mRNA stability could also be regulated by a common interaction between SOD1 and TDP-43 [34]. The exact mechanism is not completely understood; however, it is hypothesized that mutant SOD1 removes TDP-43 from the NFL mRNA, thus disturbing NFL mRNA metabolism and promoting the formation of aggregates.

In 2011, the large GGGGCC hexanucleotide repeat expansion of **C9orf72** has been recognized as a new cause of ALS [35, 36], accounting for about 50% of fALS and 5–10% of sALS [37]. The C9orf72 repeat expansion is transcribed in both the sense and antisense directions and causes the accumulations of repeat containing RNA foci [38]. RNA foci formation allows the recruitment of RBPs and alter RNA metabolism [39]. Mori and co-authors observed that RNA foci can sequester the RBP hnRNP-A3 and can suppress its RNA processing function. Notably, RNA foci are also able to sequester nuclear proteins such as TDP-43 and FUS, thus affecting the expression of their RNA targets, mainly involved in RNA metabolism, stress response, and nuclear transport. Moreover, RNA-Seq data unveil new candidate genes, that is, genes involved in synaptic transmission, protein targeting, and cell–cell signaling; however future validation are required [40]. Moreover, poly-PR and poly-GR can alter the splicing patterns of specific RNAs. The poly-PR causes the exon skipping in RAN and PTX3 RNA [41]. Finally, C9orf72 repeats can interfere with transcription or splicing of C9orf72 transcripts and can disrupt the C9orf72 promoter activity [42, 43].

3. Dysfunctions in RNA metabolism and miRNA

miRNAs are short noncoding RNAs, approximately 18–25 nucleotides long, that play a key role in the regulation of gene expression in many fundamental cellular processes and, posttranscriptionally, at the translation levels of target mRNA transcripts [44, 45]. A high number of protein-coding genes have been demonstrated to be regulated by miRNA through base-pairing interactions within the UTR of the targeted mRNAs [46, 47]. Alongside their gene silencing functions, miRNAs can also induce upregulation of their targets [48]. An accurate regulatory pathway is fundamental to control and maintain the physiological processes of cells. However, when abnormalities occur, as in diseases, a complex dysregulation of the miRNA expression takes place. In this paragraph, we will focus on miRNAs which are linked to the development of ALS and miRNA with a potential role as biomarkers.

One of the most interesting miRNAs involved in ALS is **miRNA206**. miRNA206 is skeletal muscle-specific, regulates myogenesis, and promotes the formation of new neuromuscular junctions [49, 50]. Generally, the miRNA206 is overexpressed in muscle fibers and in serum of ALS patients [50, 51]. Pegoraro and co-authors associated the high levels of miRNA206 to the remodeling of the muscle, that is, atrophy, hypertrophy, and/or reinnervation of some fibers [51]. de Andrade et al. evidenced that miRNA206 increases early in the disease course and then decreases, thus suggesting its role during muscle loss [50]. miRNAs might also have a protective role in ALS; higher levels of miRNA206 were indeed observed in slow progressors, that is, in long-term ALS patients [52]. Thanks to the possibility to detect miRNA206 in accessible samples like serum and the correlation between miRNA206 levels and disease characteristics, miRNA206 could be indicated as a potential biomarker for ALS [53]. Other three miRNAs, miRNA133a/b, miRNA 1, and miRNA 27a, are indicated as muscle-specific. **miRNA133** is higher in serum and muscle of ALS patients, and it is also higher in spinal ALS compared to bulbar ALS [51, 54]. An upregulation of **miRNA27a** was observed in CD14+ CD16− monocytes, in muscle fibers, and in CSF of ALS patients [51, 55], while a downregulation was reported in serum samples [54]. **miRNA338-3p** is another miRNA frequently upregulated. An increase of more than twofold was reported in leukocytes of sALS patients [56, 57]. Moreover, De Felice and co-authors showed an increase in miRNA338-3p in serum, CSF, and spinal cord of sALS patients. The evidence that it can be easily obtainable in body fluids suggested the possibility that miRNA338-3p might be a suitable biomarker for ALS. The inflammatory **miRNA146a** is overexpressed in CD14+ CD16− monocytes, CSF, spinal cord, and muscle fibers [55, 58]. miRNA146a can also interact with NFL mRNA 3′UTR, according to low mRNA levels observed in spinal neurons of sALS [58]. Tasca and co-authors, on the other hand, identified a reduction of miRNA146a in serum of ALS patients, both bulbar and spinal [54]. Tasca et al. and Pegoraro et al. found a downregulation in serum, muscle fibers, and leukocytes of sALS of the inflammatory **miRNA149/149***. Also **miRNA221** seems to contribute to ALS development by acting on muscle growth and/or atrophy and inflammation, through the NF-kB pathway [53, 54]. **miRNA155** was evaluated in CD14+ CD16− monocytes [55] and spinal cords of ALS patients, and it increases both in fALS and sALS [59]. Two other miRNAs targeting TGF-β1, **miRNA21,** and **miRNA106b** were upregulated in CD14+ CD16− monocytes [55], and, at least for miRNA21, an upregulation was reported in muscle samples [50] in ALS patients even if its role in the pathology has yet to be fully explained. The same authors identified an inverse correlation between **miRNA424** levels and disease progression, thus suggesting miRNA 424 as a potential biomarker [50] (**Figure 1**). The ALS genes, TDP-43 and FUS, play a role in miRNA biogenesis [60]. Mutations in TARDBP result in differential expression of **miRNA9**, **miRNA132**, **miRNA143**, **miRNA558** [61], and **let7** families [53], and differences between CSF and serum levels were observed. For instance, miRNA9, a brain-specific miRNA highly conserved during evolution is 2–3 times more elevated in CSF with respect to serum [62]. Differences are reported also for the presence of mutations. In induced pluripotent stem cell (iPSC)-derived neuron obtained from patients carrying the TARDBP p.A90V and the M337 V mutation, miRNA9 and pri-miRNA9-2 levels were lower when compared to controls [61]). Likewise, miRNA9 also decreases in lumbar motor neurons of sALS and SOD1 A4V mutated patients [63]. Moreover, a correlation between these miRNAs and disease duration and site of onset was identified. Specifically, **miRNA 143-3p** levels increase in later-collected samples, and the increase becomes significant in lower limb-onset patients [53] (**Figure 2**).

Morlando and co-authors reported that, upon FUS depletion, the expression of **miRNA9**, **miRNA132**, **miRNA143**, **miRNA125**, and **miRNA192** is altered [30]. The involvement of these miRNAs in motor neuron development and maintenance, axonal growth, and synaptic transmission accounts for their contribution to the ALS

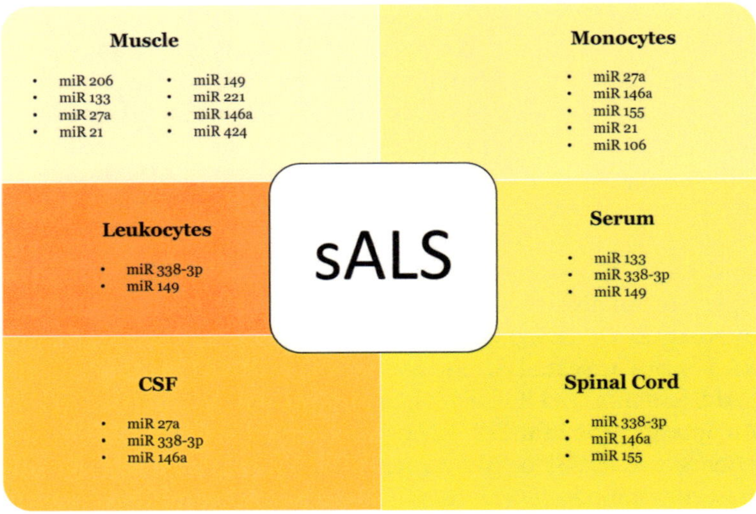

Figure 1.
Representation of the key miRNAs involved in amyotrophic lateral sclerosis sporadic patients (sALS).

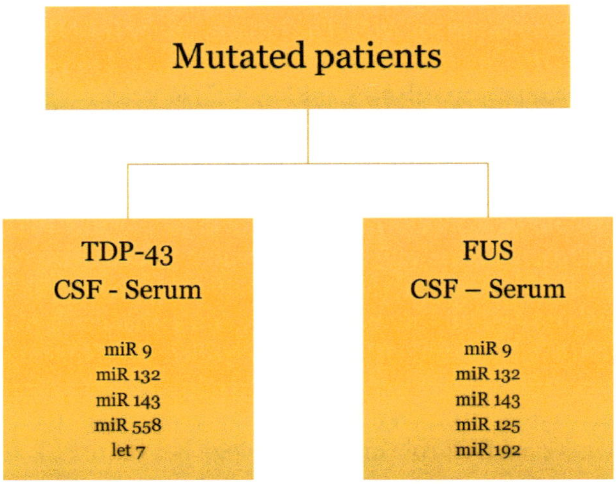

Figure 2.
Representation of the key miRNAs involved in amyotrophic lateral sclerosis mutated patients.

pathological phenotype [64, 65]. In motor neurons progenitors derived from human ALS iPSCs, Rizzuti et al. observed that **miRNA34a** and **miRNA504**, involved in vesicle regulation and cell survival, were dysregulated [66]. Also **miRNA1825** is downregulated in CNS of sALS and fALS patients, thus inducing depolymerization and degradation of tubulin alpha-4A (TUBA4A), which is encoded by the known ALS gene [67].

Taken together, these studies significantly contribute to evidence the importance of miRNAs, also as biomarkers for ALS. Despite these evidences, several issues need to be addressed mainly on the utility of miRNAs to serve as accurate and fast biomarkers for an early ALS diagnosis.

4. Dysfunctions in RNA metabolism and lncRNA

Long noncoding RNAs (lncRNAs) are transcripts, greater than 200 nucleotides in length, with no protein-coding potential which are found in sense or antisense orientation to protein-coding genes or within intergenic regions. lncRNAs control the gene expression through different mechanisms, that is, epigenetic modulation through chromatin remodeling, activation or repression of transcription, posttranscriptional modifications of mRNA, and regulation of protein activity by acting as scaffold to recruit RBPs and/or drive RBPs to DNA. Moreover, they can compete for and disrupt protein-binding interactions or sponge miRNAs away from their mRNA targets [68]. Recently, lncRNAs have been indicated to play important roles in the CNS in health and disease such as ALS. Nishimoto and colleagues first identify a relation between **NEAT1** and ALS pathogeneses [22]. The NEAT1 gene produces two transcripts, NEAT1_1 and NEAT1_2; NEAT1_2 expression is very low in the adult nervous system, and it is the only one that forms paraspeckles [69]. Specifically, NEAT1 acts as a scaffold for paraspeckles thus enhancing their de novo formation in spinal motor neurons in a cohort of sALS patients [22]. Paraspeckles function through the retention of specific RNAs; the regulation of gene expression by sequestration of transcription factors; and the modulation of miRNA biogenesis and mitochondrial function [70]. Paraspeckles are enriched in pathological proteins for ALS and are indicated as a hallmark of the disease [71]. Moreover, paraspeckle proteins, including TDP-43 and FUS, are related to ALS and FTD. The increase in paraspeckle formation in ALS could be triggered, at least in part, by the nuclear depletion of TDP-43. TDP-43 binds NEAT1, and, in turn, its downregulation stimulates NEAT1_2 accumulation and paraspeckle association in cultured cells [71]. Regarding FUS, in the spinal cord of FUS mutated ALS patients, Shelkovnikova and co-authors reported the presence of pathological aggregation of NONO, a core paraspeckle protein [31]. This evidence allows to speculate that, considering that FUS and NONO are both required to set up paraspeckles, the formation of paraspeckles is disrupted in FUS mutated ALS patients. Also aberrant nuclear RNA foci formed by the expanded C9ORF72 repeats sequester paraspeckle proteins including TDP-43 [72]. **MALAT1** is abundantly expressed and evolutionarily conserved lncRNA. It is one of the first lncRNAs associated with human disease, and it is involved in alternative splicing, epigenetic modification of gene expression, synapse formation, and myogenesis. In NDs MALAT1 is significantly increased in FTLD patients, where it recruits splicing factors to nuclear speckles and affects phosphorylation of SR proteins37 [13]. Some lncRNA transcripts have been associated to FUS, among these the **lncRNA CCND1** which binds to the FUS consensus sequence GGUG [73]. Data form Wang and colleagues suggested that FUS is a specific repressor of CCND1, which is downregulated in response to DNA damage signals. Until now the lncRNA CCND1 has not been described in relation to ALS; but taken together, these observations point out that this lncRNA could be, at least partly, responsible in ALS and other neurodegenerative diseases.

Together with the lncRNA an increasing interest was addressed to the antisense (AS) noncoding transcripts. They are generated from the strand opposite the sense strand [74]. AS lncRNAs act by regulating chromatin, by controlling DNA methylation and/or histones modification, or by removing repressors. They promote sense transcription by recruiting transcription factors, they also regulate the half-life of their sense partners, and, in turn, they regulate gene expression [74]. About 70% of the human genome creates antisense transcripts with a great physiological and pathological significance. Ataxin 2 (ATXN2) is a coding gene related to ALS because of the association between the length of ATXN2 repeat expansion and the disease risk of ALS [75]. In 2016, Li and co-authors described the **ATXN2-AS** [76]. ATXN2-AS with its CUG repeat expansion is neurotoxic and may contribute to ALS pathogenesis. The CUG transcript toxicity is related to the structure formed by the repeats; that is, the stems of hairpin structures act with sponge-like features, sequester RBPs, and induce alterations of the RNA metabolism [77].

sALS	TARDBP mutation	FUS mutation
ATXN2-AS [76]	NEAT1 [22, 69–71]	lncCCND1 [73]
ZEB1-AS [80]	MALAT1 [13]	
ZBTB11-AS [80]		
UBXN7-AS [80]		
ATG10-AS [80]		
ADORA2A-AS [80]		

Table 1.
List of lncRNAs related to ALS. In square bracket the relative references.

Thanks to the deep sequencing technologies which allow high-throughput massive RNA sequencing, a wide characterization of the transcriptome profile of cell populations and tissues is now available. Three different massive transcriptome profiles have been published in different tissues (spinal cord, monocytes, and peripheral blood mononuclear cells) of ALS patients, and matched controls reported a deregulation in expressed genes [78, 79] and in lncRNAs [80]. Differences in transcriptome profiles (coding and lncRNAs) were observed in PBMCs of unmutated sALS patients, SOD1, TARDBP, and FUS mutated ALS patients and healthy controls [80]. Specifically, the authors reported a remarkable AS deregulation of genes involved in the transcription regulation pathway such as **ZEB1-AS** and **ZBTB11-AS** in sALS patients. ZEB1 acts as a repressor or an activator of the transcription, that is, it may repress histone organization or activate chromatin regulators [81]. As regards ZBTB11-AS, it decreases in sALS patients compared to healthy controls. ZBTB11-AS is annotated as AS of Zinc finger and BTB domain-containing protein 11 (ZBTB11) gene, and it is reported to be a negative regulator of cell cycle; however its exact role has yet to be defined [82]. Moreover, Gagliardi and co-authors evidenced **UBXN7-AS**, **ATG10-AS,** and **ADORA2A-AS** in sALS patients, all related to NDs [83–85]. Specifically, the regulation of UBXN7, an ubiquitin protein bound by VCP a known ALS protein, through its AS controlled the ubiquitination in ALS disease. ATG10 is involved in the autophagy pathway, while ADORA2A is involved in Huntington's disease and Parkinson's disease in relation to defects in DNA methylation [84, 86] (**Table 1**).

5. Therapeutics

In the era of noncoding RNA, understanding the involvement of dysregulated miRNAs and of their targets in ALS disease is crucial to identify new pathways contributing to neurodegeneration that also offer novel opportunities for targeted intervention. miRNA-based therapeutics take advantages of two different approaches. The first involves the use of an anti-miRNA, that is, chemically modified antisense RNA, to decrease miRNA. Thus, miRNA duplex is not active and counteracts the negative regulatory effects of miRNA. This approach was first used to deliver the anti-miR-155 to the SOD1G93A transgenic mice via ventricular osmotic pumps; after this treatment the mortality was successfully delayed [59]. The second therapeutic approach using miRNA involves miRNA mimics, that is, small RNA molecules resembling miRNA precursors, that are reintroduced into cells exhibiting downregulation thus re-starting the key-related pathways [87]. Biomedical and nanoparticle engineering has begun to develop tools allowing for this specific targeting. These second-generation miRNA-based therapeutics offer the potential for a greater delivery cargo to the tissue site while reducing RNA-mediated toxicity. Overall, the continued development of innovative RNA modifications and delivery items such as nanoparticles will aid in the development of future RNA-based therapeutics for a broader range of chronic disease.

Deregulated AS is considered an important area for therapeutic intervention. Particularly, gene therapy is an encouraging pharmacological approach for patients with diseases of genetic origins. This therapy is principally based on antisense oligonucleotides (ASOs), spliceosome-mediated RNA trans-splicing (SMaRT), or small interfering RNAs (siRNAs) [88]. ASOs, that is, synthetic single-stranded nucleic acids, bind the pre-mRNA intron/exon junctions and control the splicing through their action on enhancers or repressor sequences, thus determining the skipping of the exon or including alternatively spliced exons [89].

In ALS, one of the first ASO-based clinical trials was designed to silence SOD1. The intrathecal administration of this ASO pass with good results the phase I testing. Now a phase Ib/IIa trial is in process to assess safety, tolerability, and pharmacokinetics [90].

Among the ALS-related genes, C9orf72 is one of the best candidates for ASOs therapy. Early testing of ASO-based therapeutics for C9orf72 was performed on iPSC-derived neurons and fibroblasts [91]. Specifically, ASOs were designed to target the repeat expansion or within N-terminal regions of the mRNA transcript to destroy the transcript or to prevent the interaction between the repeat expansion and the RBPs, determining a decrease in RNA foci and dipeptide proteins and recovering the normal gene expression [91]. Other studies investigated the effects of ASO on the oligonucleotide backbone, sugar, and heterocycles to promote delivery, potency, and stability to target FUS. These studies evidenced that the affinities of nucleic acid binding domains depend on chemical changes and that the interaction between ASO and protein affects the localization of ASOs themselves [92]. These data strongly indicate that ASO-based therapy could be central in treating ALS-related genes, although there is great attention on the relation between the therapeutic outcomes and the stage of disease progression and on the time of intervention.

Also many novel lncRNAs have been discovered, and the potential to become therapeutic targets is gradually increasing. Considering that lncRNAs function as decoys, regulators of translation, and scaffolds directing chromatin-modifying enzymes to specific genomic loci, they are an attractive class of therapeutic targets. The relation between HOTAIR in breast cancer [93] and MALAT1 in metastatic lung cancer [94] is a remarkable example of this association. Therefore, there is enthusiasm about the possibility to develop therapeutic tools to modulate mis-regulated lncRNAs in diseases. Although lncRNAs represent appealing pharmacological and therapeutic targets, inhibiting lncRNAs in vivo remains a challenge. A possible approach could be the use of small molecules that disrupt the complex lncRNA-chromatin that alter the epigenetic state of the target cells. All these delivery efforts, along with further elucidation of lncRNA regulatory mechanisms, will ultimately lead to the development of effective therapeutic strategies that target lncRNAs in vivo.

6. Conclusion

The impairment in RNA regulation and processing is crucial in ALS pathogenesis. Defects at different steps of RNA processing alter both cellular function and survival; thus RNA metabolism can be an essential target for therapeutic intervention for ALS and for other NDs. The application of RNA-based therapies to modulate gene and protein expression is an interesting therapeutic strategy:

the preclinical application of RNA-based therapies targeting SOD1 and C9orf72 mutations are promising and pave the way to apply similar approaches for FUS and TDP-43 mutations. In conclusion, RNA-based therapies could be recommended for the future treatment of ALS.

Funding

Authors acknowledge the economic support of the Fondazione Regionale per la Ricerca Biomedica (FRRB): TRANS_ALS [2015-0023]; Finanziamento 5x1000 2016; Italian Ministry of Health GR-2016-02361552.

Abbreviations

ABLIM1	actin-binding LIM
ADORA2A	adenosine A2a receptor
ALS	amyotrophic lateral sclerosis
ANG	angiogenin
ANXA11	annexin A11
AS	antisense
ASOs	antisense oligonucleotides
ATG10	autophagy related 10
ATXN2	ataxin 2
C9ORF72	chromosome 9 open reading frame 72
CCND1	cyclin D1
CHCHD10	coiled-coil-helix-coiled-coil-helix domain containing 10
CHMP2B	charged multivesicular body protein 2B
CNS	central nervous system
CSF	cerebrospinal fluid
EWSR1	EWS RNA binding protein 1
fALS	familial amyotrophic lateral sclerosis
FTLD	frontotemporal lobar degeneration
FUS	fused in sarcoma/translocated in liposarcoma
GABRA2	gamma-aminobutyric acid type A receptor alpha2 subunit
GABRA3	gamma-aminobutyric acid type A receptor alpha3 subunit
GRIA3	glutamate ionotropic receptor AMPA type subunit 3AMPA receptor subunits
GRIA4	glutamate ionotropic receptor AMPA type subunit 4AMPA receptor subunits
HNRNPA1	heterogeneous nuclear ribonucleoprotein A1
HNRNPA2/B1	heterogeneous nuclear ribonucleoprotein A2/B1
Homer2	homer scaffold protein 2
HOTAIR	HOX transcript antisense RNA
HuR	Hu antigen R
iPSC	induced pluripotent stem cell
KIF5A	kinesin family member 5A
lncRNA	long noncoding RNA
lncRNAs	long noncoding RNAs
MALAT1	metastasis-associated lung adenocarcinoma transcript 1
MAP1B	microtubule-associated protein 1B
MAPT	microtubule-associated protein tau
MATR3	matrin 3

miRNAs	microRNAs
MN	motor neuron
ND	neurodegenerative disorder
NEAT1	nuclear-enriched autosomal transcript 1
NES	nuclear export signals
NF-kB	nuclear factor kappa B subunit 1
NFL	neurofilament light chain
NLGN1-2	neuroligin
NLS	nuclear localization
NONO	non-POU domain-containing octamer-binding protein
NRCAM	neuronal cell adhesion molecule
NRXN1-3	neurexin
NTNG1	netrin G1
OPTN	optineurin
PFN1	profilin 1
PTX3	pentraxin 3
RBP	RNA-binding proteins
RRM1-2	RNA recognition motifs 1-2
RUNX	Runbox transcription factor
sALS	sporadic amyotrophic lateral sclerosis
siRNAs	small interfering RNAs
SMaRT	spliceosome-mediated RNA trans-splicing
SOD1	superoxide dismutase 1
SPI1	Spi-1 proto-oncogene
SQSTM1	sequestosome 1
SYGQ	N-terminal serine-tyrosine-glycine-glutamine
TAF15	TATA-box binding protein-associated factor 15
TARDBP	TAR DNA-binding protein
TBK1	TANK-binding kinase 1
TGF-β1	transforming growth factor-beta
TIAR	TIA1 cytotoxic granule-associated RNA binding protein like 1
TUBA4A	tubulin alpha 4a
UBQLN2	ubiquilin 1
UBXN7	UBX domain protein 7
UTR	3′-untranslated
VAPB	vesicle-associated membrane protein-associated protein B/C
VCP	valosin-containing protein
VEGF	vascular endothelial growth factor
ZBTB11	zinc finger and BTB domain-containing 11
ZEB1	zinc finger E-box-binding homeobox 1

Author details

Orietta Pansarasa*, Stella Gagliardi, Daisy Sproviero and Cristina Cereda
Genomic and Post-Genomic Center, IRCCS Mondino Foundation, Pavia, Italy

*Address all correspondence to: orietta.pansarasa@mondino.it

References

[1] Kiernan MC, Vucic S, Cheah BC, Turner MR, Eisen A, Hardiman O, et al. Amyotrophic lateral sclerosis. Lancet. 2011;**377**(9769):942-955. DOI: 10.1016/S0140-6736(10)61156-7

[2] Hardiman O, Al-Chalabi A, Chio A, Corr EM, Logroscino G, Robberecht W, et al. Amyotrophic lateral sclerosis. Nature Reviews. Disease Primers. 2017;**3**:17071. DOI: 10.1038/nrdp.2017.71

[3] Nguyen HP, Van Broeckhoven C, van der Zee J. ALS genes in the genomic era and their implications for FTD. Trends in Genetics. 2018;**34**(6):404-423. DOI: 10.1016/j.tig.2018.03.001

[4] Taylor JP, Brown RH Jr, Cleveland DW. Decoding ALS: From genes to mechanism. Nature. 2016;**539**(7628):197-206. DOI: 10.1038/nature20413

[5] Cook C, Petrucelli L. Genetic convergence brings clarity to the enigmatic red line in ALS. Neuron. 2019;**101**(6):1057-1069. DOI: 10.1016/j.neuron.2019.02.032

[6] Sicot G, Gomes-Pereira M. RNA toxicity in human disease and animal models: From the uncovering of a new mechanism to the development of promising therapies. Biochimica et Biophysica Acta. 2013;**1832**(9):1390-1409. DOI: 10.1016/j.bbadis.2013.03.002

[7] Nussbacher JK, Batra R, Lagier-Tourenne C, Yeo GW. RNA-binding proteins in neurodegeneration: Seq and you shall receive. Trends in Neurosciences. 2015;**38**(4):226-236. DOI: 10.1016/j.tins.2015.02.003

[8] Buratti E, Baralle FE. Characterization and functional implications of the RNA binding properties of nuclear factor TDP-43, a novel splicing regulator of CFTR exon 9. The Journal of Biological Chemistry. 2001;**76**:36337-36343. DOI: 10.1074/jbc. M104236200

[9] Winton MJ, Igaz LM, Wong MM, Kwong LK, Trojanowski JQ, Lee VM. Disturbance of nuclear and cytoplasmic TAR DNA-binding protein (TDP-43) induces disease-like redistribution, sequestration, and aggregate formation. The Journal of Biological Chemistry. 2008;**283**:13302-13309. DOI: 10.1074/jbc.M800342200

[10] Buratti E, Baralle FE. Multiple roles of TDP-43 in gene expression, splicing regulation, and human disease. Frontiers in Bioscience. 2008;**13**:867-878. DOI: 10.2741/2727

[11] Polymenidou M, Lagier-Tourenne C, Hutt KR, Huelga SC, Moran J, Liang TY, et al. Long pre-mRNA depletion and RNA missplicing contribute to neuronal vulnerability from loss of TDP-43. Nature Neuroscience. 2011;**14**:459-468. DOI: 10.1038/nn.2779

[12] Colombrita C, Onesto E, Megiorni F, Pizzuti A, Baralle FE, Buratti E, et al. TDP-43 and FUS RNA-binding proteins bind distinct sets of cytoplasmic messenger RNAs and differently regulate their post-transcriptional fate in motoneuron-like cells. The Journal of Biological Chemistry. 2012;**287**:15635-15647. DOI: 10.1074/jbc.M111.333450

[13] Tollervey JR, Curk T, Rogelj B, Briese M, Cereda M, Kayikci M, et al. Characterizing the RNA targets and position-dependent splicing regulation by TDP-43. Nature Neuroscience. 2011;**14**:452-458. DOI: 10.1038/nn.2778

[14] Sephton CF, Cenik C, Kucukural A, Dammer EB, Cenik B, Han Y, et al. Identification of neuronal RNA targets of TDP-43-containing ribonucleoprotein complexes. The Journal of Biological Chemistry. 2011;**286**:1204-1215. DOI: 10.1074/jbc. M110.190884

[15] Narayanan RK, Mangelsdorf M, Panwar A, Butler TJ, Noakes PG,

Wallace RH. Identification of RNA bound to the TDP-43 ribonucleoprotein complex in the adult mouse brain. Amyotrophic Lateral Sclerosis and Frontotemporal Degeneration. 2013;**14**:252-260. DOI: 10.3109/21678421.2012.734520

[16] Chang JC, Hazelett DJ, Stewart JA, Morton DB. Motor neuron expression of the voltage-gated calcium channel cacophony restores locomotion defects in a drosophila, TDP-43 loss of function model of ALS. Brain Research. 2014;**1584**:39-51. DOI: 10.1016/j.brainres.2013.11.019

[17] Coyne AN, Siddegowda BB, Estes PS, Johannesmeyer J, Kovalik T, Daniel SG, et al. Futsch/MAP1B mRNA is a translational target of TDP-43 and is neuroprotective in a drosophila model of amyotrophic lateral sclerosis. The Journal of Neuroscience. 2014;**34**:15962-15974. DOI: 10.1523/JNEUROSCI.2526-14.2014

[18] Ayala YM, De Conti L, Avendaño-Vázquez SE, Dhir A, Romano M, D'Ambrogio A, et al. TDP-43 regulates its mRNA levels through a negative feedback loop. The EMBO Journal. 2011;**30**:277-288. DOI: 10.1038/emboj.2010.310

[19] Yang C, Wang H, Qiao T, Yang B, Aliaga L, Qiu L, et al. Partial loss of TDP-43 function causes phenotypes of amyotrophic lateral sclerosis. Proceedings of the National Academy of Sciences of the United States of America. 2014;**111**:E1121-E1129. DOI: 10.1073/pnas.1322641111

[20] Kawahara Y, Mieda-Sato A. TDP-43 promotes microRNA biogenesis as a component of the Drosha and dicer complexes. Proceedings of the National Academy of Sciences of the United States of America. 2012;**109**(9):3347-3352. DOI: 10.1073/pnas.1112427109

[21] Buratti E, De Conti L, Stuani C, Romano M, Baralle M, Baralle F. Nuclear factor TDP-43 can affect selected microRNA levels. The FEBS Journal. 2010;**277**:2268-2281. DOI: 10.1111/j.1742-4658.2010.07643.x

[22] Nishimoto Y, Nakagawa S, Hirose T, Okano HJ, Takao M, Shibata S, et al. The long non-coding RNA nuclear-enriched abundant transcript 1_2 induces paraspeckle formation in the motor neuron during the early phase of amyotrophic lateral sclerosis. Molecular Brain. 2013;**6**:31. DOI: 10.1186/1756-6606-6-31

[23] Iko Y, Kodama TS, Kasai N, Oyama T, Morita EH, Muto T, et al. Domainarchitecturesandcharacterization of an RNA-binding protein, TLS. The Journal of Biological Chemistry. 2004;**279**:44834-44840. DOI: 10.1074/jbc.M408552200

[24] Uranishi H, Tetsuka T, Yamashita M, Asamitsu K, Shimizu M, Itoh M, et al. Involvement of the pro-oncoprotein TLS (translocated in liposarcoma) in nuclear factor-k B p65-mediated transcription as a coactivator. The Journal of Biological Chemistry. 2001;**276**:13395-13401. DOI: 10.1074/jbc.M011176200

[25] Li X, Decker M, Westendorf JJ. TEThered to Runx: Novel binding partners for runx factors. Blood Cells, Molecules & Diseases. 2010;**45**:82-85. DOI: 10.1016/j.bcmd.2010.03.002

[26] Lagier-Tourenne C, Polymenidou M, Hutt KR, Vu AQ, Baughn M, Huelga SC, et al. Divergent roles of ALS-linked proteins FUS/TLS and TDP-43 intersect in processing long pre-mRNAs. Nature Neuroscience. 2012;**15**:1488-1497. DOI: 10.1038/nn.3230

[27] Ishigaki S, Masuda A, Fujioka Y, Iguchi Y, Katsuno M, Shibata A, et al. Position-dependent FUS-RNA interactions regulate alternative splicing

events and transcriptions. Scientific Reports. 2012;**2**:529. DOI: 10.1038/srep00529

[28] Rogelj B, Easton LE, Bogu GK, Stanton LW, Rot G, Curk T, et al. Widespread binding of FUS along nascent RNA regulates alternative splicing in the brain. Scientific Reports. 2012;**2**:603. DOI: 10.1038/srep00603

[29] Nakaya T, Alexiou P, Maragkakis M, Chang A, Mourelatos Z. FUS regulates genes coding for RNA-binding proteins in neurons by binding to their highly conserved introns. RNA. 2013;**19**:498-509. DOI: 10.1261/rna.037804.112

[30] Morlando M, Dini Modigliani S, Torrelli G, Rosa A, Di Carlo V, Caffarelli E, et al. FUS stimulates microRNA biogenesis by facilitating co-transcriptional Drosha recruitment. The EMBO Journal. 2012;**31**:4502-4510. DOI: 10.1038/emboj.2012.319

[31] Shelkovnikova TA, Robinson HK, Troakes C, Ninkina N, Buchman VL. Compromised paraspeckle formation as a pathogenic factor in FUSopathies. Human Molecular Genetics. 2014;**23**(9):2298-2312. DOI: 10.1093/hmg/ddt622

[32] Lu L, Wang S, Zheng L, Li X, Suswam EA, Zhang X, et al. Amyotrophic lateral sclerosis-linked mutant SOD1 sequesters Hu antigen R (HuR) and TIA-1-related protein (TIAR): Implications for impaired posttranscriptional regulation of vascular endothelial growth factor. The Journal of Biological Chemistry. 2009;**284**:33989-33998. DOI: 10.1074/jbc.M109.067918

[33] Chen H, Qian K, Du Z, Cao J, Petersen A, Liu H, et al. Modeling ALS with iPSCs reveals that mutant SOD1 misregulates neurofilament balance in motor neurons. Cell Stem Cell. 2014;**14**:796-809. DOI: 10.1016/j.stem.2014.02.004

[34] Volkening K, Leystra-Lantz C, Yang W, Jaffee H, Strong MJ. Tar DNA binding protein of 43 kDa (TDP-43), 14-3-3 proteins and copper/zinc superoxide dismutase (SOD1) interact to modulate NFL mRNA stability. Implications for altered RNA processing in amyotrophic lateral sclerosis (ALS). Brain Research. 2009;**1305**:168-182. DOI: 10.1016/j.brainres.2009.09.105

[35] De Jesus-Hernandez M, Mackenzie IR, Boeve BF, Boxer AL, Baker M, Rutherford NJ, et al. Expanded GGGGCC hexanucleotide repeat in noncoding region of C9ORF72 causes chromosome 9p-linked FTD and ALS. Neuron. 2011;**72**:245-256. DOI: 10.1016/j.neuron.2011.09.011

[36] Renton AE, Majounie E, Waite A, Simón-Sánchez J, Rollinson S, Gibbs JR, et al. A hexanucleotide repeat expansion in C9ORF72 is the cause of chromosome 9p21-linked ALS-FTD. Neuron. 2011;**72**:257-268. DOI: 10.1016/j.neuron.2011.09.010

[37] Majounie E, Renton AE, Mok K, Dopper EG, Waite A, Rollinson S, et al. Frequency of the C9orf72 hexanucleotide repeat expansion in patients with amyotrophic lateral sclerosis and frontotemporal dementia: A cross-sectional study. Lancet Neurology. 2012;**11**:323-330. DOI: 10.1016/S1474-4422(12) 70043-1

[38] Gendron TF, Bieniek KF, Zhang YJ, Jansen-West K, Ash PE, Caulfield T, et al. Antisense transcripts of the expanded C9ORF72 hexanucleotide repeat form nuclear RNA foci and undergo repeat-associated non-ATG translation in c9FTD/ALS. Acta Neuropathologica. 2013;**126**:829-844. DOI: 10.1007/s00401-013-1192-8

[39] Mori K, Lammich S, Mackenzie IR, Forné I, Zilow S, Kretzschmar H, et al. hnRNP A3 binds to GGGGCC repeats

and is a constituent of p62-positive/TDP43-negative inclusions in the hippocampus of patients with C9orf72 mutations. Acta Neuropathologica. 2013a;**125**:413-423. DOI: 10.1007/s00401-013-1088-7

[40] Selvaraj BT, Livesey MR, Zhao C, Gregory JM, James OT, Cleary EM, et al. C9ORF72 repeat expansion causes vulnerability of motor neurons to Ca2C-permeable AMPA receptor-mediated excitotoxicity. Nature Communications. 2018;**9**:347. DOI: 10.1038/s41467-017-02729-0

[41] Kwon I, Xiang S, Kato M, Wu L, Theodoropoulos P, Wang T, et al. Poly-dipeptides encoded by the C9orf72 repeats bind nucleoli, impede RNA biogenesis, and kill cells. Science. 2014;**345**:1139-1145. DOI: 10.1126/science.1254917

[42] Mori K, Weng SM, Arzberger T, May S, Rentzsch K, Kremmer E, et al. The C9orf72 GGGGCC repeat is translated into aggregating dipeptiderepeat proteins in FTLD/ALS. Science. 2013b;**339**:1335-1338. DOI: 10.1126/science.1232927

[43] Gijselinck I, Van Mossevelde S, van der Zee J, Sieben A, Engelborghs S, De Bleecker J, et al. The C9orf72 repeat size correlates with onset age of disease, DNA methylation and transcriptional downregulation of the promoter. Molecular Psychiatry. 2016;**21**:1112-1124. DOI: 10.1038/mp.2015.159

[44] Quinlan S, Kenny A, Medina M, Engel T, Jimenez-Mateos EM. MicroRNAs in neurodegenerative diseases. International Review of Cell and Molecular Biology. 2017;**334**:309-343. DOI: 10.1016/bs.ircmb.2017.04.002

[45] Krokidis MG, Vlamos P. Transcriptomics in amyotrophic lateral sclerosis. Frontiers in Bioscience. 2018;**10**:103-121

[46] Roshan R, Ghosh T, Scaria V, Pillai B. MicroRNAs: Novel therapeutic targets in neurodegenerative diseases. Drug Discovery Today. 2009;**14**(23-24):1123-1129. DOI: 10.1016/j.drudis.2009.09.009

[47] Cloutier F, Marrero A, O'Connell C, Morin P Jr. MicroRNAs as potential circulating biomarkers for amyotrophic lateral sclerosis. Journal of Molecular Neuroscience. 2015;**56**(1):102-112. DOI: 10.1007/s12031-014-0471-8

[48] Vasudevan S, Tong Y, Steitz JA. Switching from repression to activation: microRNAs can up-regulate translation. Science. 2007;**318**:1931-1934. DOI: 10.1126/science.1149460

[49] Goljanek-Whysall K, Pais H, Rathjen T, Sweetman D, Dalmay T, Munsterberg A. Regulation of multiple target genes by miR-1 and miR-206 is pivotal for C2C12 myoblast differentiation. Journal of Cell Science. 2012;**125**:3590-3600. DOI: 10.1242/jcs.101758

[50] de Andrade HM, de Albuquerque M, Avansini SH, de S Rocha C, Dogini DB, Nucci A, et al. MicroRNAs-424 and 206 are potential prognostic markers in spinal onset amyotrophic lateral sclerosis. Journal of the Neurological Sciences. 2016;**368**:19-24. DOI: 10.1016/j.jns.2016.06.046

[51] Pegoraro V, Merico A, Angelini C. Micro-RNAs in ALS muscle: Differences in gender, age at onset and disease duration. Journal of the Neurological Sciences. 2017;**380**:58-63. DOI: 10.1016/j.jns.2017.07.008

[52] Bruneteau G, Simonet T, Bauché S, Mandjee N, Malfatti E, Girard E, et al. Muscle histone deacetylase 4 upregulation in amyotrophic lateral sclerosis: Potential role in reinnervation ability and disease progression. Brain. 2013;**136**(Pt 8):2359-2368. DOI: 10.1093/brain/awt164

[53] Waller R, Goodall EF, Milo M, Cooper-Knock J, Da Costa M, Hobson E, et al. Serum miRNAs miR-206, 143-3p and 374b-5p as potential biomarkers for amyotrophic lateral sclerosis (ALS). Neurobiology of Aging. 2017;**55**:123-131. DOI: 10.1016/j.neurobiolaging.2017.03.027

[54] Tasca E, Pegoraro V, Merico A, Angelini C. Circulating microRNAs as biomarkers of muscle differentiation and atrophy in ALS. Clinical Neuropathology. 2016;**35**:22-30. DOI: 10.5414/ np300889

[55] Butovsky O, Siddiqui S, Gabriely G, Lanser AJ, Dake B, Murugaiyan G, et al. Modulating inflammatory monocytes with a unique microRNA gene signature ameliorates murine ALS. The Journal of Clinical Investigation. 2012;**122**(9):3063-3087. DOI: 10.1172/JCI62636

[56] De Felice B, Guida M, Guida M, Coppola C, De Mieri G, Cotrufo R. A miRNA signature in leukocytes from sporadic amyotrophic lateral sclerosis. Gene. 2012;**508**:35-40. DOI: 10.1016/j.gene.2012.07.058

[57] De Felice B, Annunziata A, Fiorentino G, Borra M, Biffali E, Coppola C, et al. miR-338-3p is over-expressed in blood, CFS, serum and spinal cord from sporadic amyotrophic lateral sclerosis patients. Neurogenetics. 2014;**15**(4):243-253. DOI: 10.1007/s10048-014-0420-2

[58] Campos-Melo D, Droppelmann CA, He Z, Volkening K, Strong MJ. Altered microRNA expression profile in amyotrophic lateral sclerosis: A role in the regulation of NFL mRNA levels. Molecular Brain. 2013;**6**:26. DOI: 10.1186/1756-6606-6-26

[59] Koval ED, Shaner C, Zhang P, du Maine X, Fischer K, Tay J, et al. Method for widespread microRNA-155 inhibition prolongs survival in ALS-model mice. Human Molecular Genetics. 2013;**22**(20):4127-4135. DOI: 10.1093/hmg/ddt261

[60] Da Cruz S, Cleveland DW. Understanding the role of TDP-43 and FUS/TLS in ALS and beyond. Current Opinion in Neurobiology. 2011;**21**:904-919. DOI: 10.1016/j.conb.2011.05.029

[61] Zhang Z, Almeida S, Lu Y, Nishimura AL, Peng L, Sun D, et al. Downregulation of microRNA-9 in iPSC-derived neurons of FTD/ALS patients with TDP-43 mutations. PLoS One. 2013;**8**(10):e76055. DOI: 10.1371/journal.pone.0076055

[62] Freischmidt A, Müller K, Ludolph AC, Weishaupt JH. Systemic dysregulation of TDP-43 binding microRNAs in amyotrophic lateral sclerosis. Acta Neuropathologica Communications. 2013;**1**:42. DOI: 10.1186/2051-5960-1-42

[63] Emde A, Eitan C, Liou LL, Libby RT, Rivkin N, Magen I, et al. Dysregulated miRNA biogenesis downstream of cellular stress and ALS-causing mutations: A new mechanism for ALS. The EMBO Journal. 2015;**34**(21):2633-2651. DOI: 10.15252/embj.201490493

[64] Luxenhofer G, Helmbrecht MS, Langhoff J, Giusti SA, Refojo D, Huber AB. MicroRNA-9 promotes the switch from early-born to late-born motor neuron populations by regulating Onecut transcription factor expression. Developmental Biology. 2014;**386**(2):358-370. DOI: 10.1016/j.ydbio.2013.12.023

[65] Edbauer D, Neilson JR, Foster KA, Wang CF, Seeburg DP, Batterton MN, et al. Regulation of synaptic structure and function by FMRP-associated microRNAs miR-125b and miR-132. Neuron. 2010;**65**(3):373-384. DOI: 10.1016/j.neuron.2010.01.005. Erratum in: Neuron. 2010;68(1):161

[66] Rizzuti M, Filosa G, Melzi V, Calandriello L, Dioni L, Bollati V, et al. MicroRNA expression analysis identifies a subset of downregulated miRNAs in ALS motor neuron progenitors. Scientific Reports. 2018;**8**(1):10105. DOI: 10.1038/s41598-018-28366-1

[67] Helferich AM, Brockmann SJ, Reinders J, Deshpande D, Holzmann K, Brenner D, et al. Dysregulation of a novel miR-1825/TBCB/TUBA4A pathway in sporadic and familial ALS. Cellular and Molecular Life Sciences. 2018;**75**(23):4301-4319. DOI: 10.1007/s00018-018-2873-1

[68] Ponting CP, Oliver PL, Reik W. Evolution and functions of long noncoding RNAs. Cell. 2009;**136**(4):629-641. DOI: 10.1016/j.cell.2009.02.006

[69] Clemson CM, Hutchinson JN, Sara SA, Ensminger AW, Fox AH, Chess A, et al. An architectural role for a nuclear noncoding RNA: NEAT1 RNA is essential for the structure of paraspeckles. Molecular Cell. 2009;**33**:717-726. DOI: 10.1016/j.molcel.2009.01.026

[70] Hirose T, Virnicchi G, Tanigawa A, Naganuma T, Li R, Kimura H, et al. NEAT1 long noncoding RNA regulates transcription via protein sequestration within subnuclear bodies. Molecular Biology of the Cell. 2014;**25**(1):169-183. DOI: 10.1091/mbc.E13-09-0558

[71] An H, Williams NG, Shelkovnikova TA. NEAT1 and paraspeckles in neurodegenerative diseases: A missing lnc found? Non-coding RNA Research. 2018;**3**(4):243-252. DOI: 10.1016/j.ncrna.2018.11.003

[72] Česnik BA, Darovic S, Prpar Mihevc S, Štalekar M, Malnar M, Motaln H, et al. Nuclear RNA foci from C9ORF72 expansion mutation form paraspeckle-like bodies. Journal of Cell Science. 2019;**132**(5):jcs224303. DOI: 10.1242/jcs.224303

[73] Wang X, Arai S, Song X, Reichart D, Du K, Pascual G, et al. Induced ncRNAs allosterically modify RNA-binding proteins in cis to inhibit transcription. Nature. 2008;**454**(7200):126-130. DOI: 10.1038/nature06992

[74] Pelechano V, Steinmetz LM. Gene regulation by antisense transcription. Nature Reviews. Genetics. 2013;**14**(12):880-893. DOI: 10.1038/nrg3594

[75] Elden AC, Kim HJ, Hart MP, Chen-Plotkin AS, Johnson BS, Fang X, et al. Ataxin-2 intermediate-length polyglutamine expansions are associated with increased risk for ALS. Nature. 2010;**466**(7310):1069-1075. DOI: 10.1038/nature09320

[76] Li PP, Sun X, Xia G, Arbez N, Paul S, Zhu S, et al. ATXN2-AS, a gene antisense to ATXN2, is associated with spinocerebellar ataxia type 2 and amyotrophic lateral sclerosis. Annals of Neurology. 2016;**80**(4):600-615. DOI: 10.1002/ana.24761

[77] Nalavade R, Griesche N, Ryan DP, Hildebrand S, Krauss S. Mechanisms of RNA-induced toxicity in CAG repeat disorders. Cell Death & Disease. 2013;**4**:e752. DOI: 10.1038/cddis.2013.276

[78] D'Erchia AM, Gallo A, Manzari C, Raho S, Horner DS, Chiara M, et al. Massive transcriptome sequencing of human spinal cord tissues provides new insights into motor neuron degeneration in ALS. Scientific Reports. 2017;**7**(1):10046. DOI: 10.1038/s41598-017-10488-7

[79] Zhao W, Beers DR, Hooten KG, Sieglaff DH, Zhang A, Kalyana-Sundaram S, et al. Characterization of gene expression phenotype in

amyotrophic lateral sclerosis monocytes. JAMA Neurology. 2017;**74**(6):677-685. DOI: 10.1001/jamaneurol.2017.0357

[80] Gagliardi S, Zucca S, Pandini C, Diamanti L, Bordoni M, Sproviero D, et al. Long non-coding and coding RNAs characterization in peripheral blood mononuclear cells and spinal cord from amyotrophic lateral sclerosis patients. Scientific Reports. 2018;**8**(1):2378. DOI: 10.1038/s41598-018-20679-5

[81] Li T, Xie J, Shen C, Cheng D, Shi Y, Wu Z, et al. Upregulation of long noncoding RNA ZEB1-AS1 promotes tumor metastasis and predicts poor prognosis in hepatocellular carcinoma. Oncogene. 2016;**35**(12):1575-1584. DOI: 10.1038/onc.2015.223

[82] Keightley MC, Carradice DP, Layton JE, Pase L, Bertrand JY, Wittig JG, et al. The Pu.1 target gene Zbtb11 regulates neutrophil development through its integrase-like HHCC zinc finger. Nature Communications. 2017;**8**:14911. DOI: 10.1038/ncomms14911

[83] Villar-Menéndez I, Porta S, Buira SP, Pereira-Veiga T, Díaz-Sánchez S, Albasanz JL, et al. Increased striatal adenosine A2A receptor levels is an early event in Parkinson's disease-related pathology and it is potentially regulated by miR-34b. Neurobiology of Disease. 2014;**69**:206-214. DOI: 10.1016/j.nbd.2014.05.030

[84] Lee JK, Shin JH, Lee JE, Choi EJ. Role of autophagy in the pathogenesis of amyotrophic lateral sclerosis. Biochimica et Biophysica Acta. 2015 Nov;**1852**(11):2517-2524. DOI: 10.1016/j.bbadis.2015.08.005

[85] Guo X, Qi X. VCP cooperates with UBXD1 to degrade mitochondrial outer membrane protein MCL1 in model of Huntington's disease. Biochimica et Biophysica Acta - Molecular Basis of Disease. 2017;**1863**(2):552-559. DOI: 10.1016/j.bbadis.2016.11.026

[86] Majidinia M, Mihanfar A, Rahbarghazi R, Nourazarian A, Bagca B, Avci ÇB. The roles of non-coding RNAs in Parkinson's disease. Molecular Biology Reports. 2016;**43**(11):1193-1204

[87] Bader AG, Brown D, Winkler M. The promise of microRNA replacement therapy. Cancer Research. 2010;**70**(18):7027-7030. DOI: 10.1158/0008-5472.CAN-10-2010

[88] Arechavala-Gomeza V, Khoo B, Aartsma-Rus A. Splicing modulation therapy in the treatment of genetic diseases. The Application of Clinical Genetics. 2014;**7**:245-252. DOI: 10.2147/TACG.S71506

[89] Havens MA, Hastings ML. Splice-switching antisense oligonucleotides as therapeutic drugs. Nucleic Acids Research. 2016;**44**(14):6549-6563. DOI: 10.1093/nar/gkw533

[90] McCampbell A, Cole T, Wegener AJ, Tomassy GS, Setnicka A, Farley BJ, et al. Antisense oligonucleotides extend survival and reverse decrement in muscle response in ALS models. The Journal of Clinical Investigation. 2018;**128**(8):3558-3567. DOI: 10.1172/JCI99081

[91] Butti Z, Patten SA. RNA Dysregulation in amyotrophic lateral sclerosis. Frontiers in Genetics. 2019;**9**:712. DOI: 10.3389/fgene.2018.00712

[92] Bailey JK, Shen W, Liang XH, Crooke ST. Nucleic acid binding proteins affect the subcellular distribution of phosphorothioate antisense oligonucleotides. Nucleic Acids Research. 2017 Oct 13;**45**(18):10649-10671. DOI: 10.1093/nar/gkx709

[93] Han B, Peng X, Cheng D, Zhu Y, Du J, Li J, et al. Delphinidin suppresses breast carcinogenesis through the HOTAIR/microRNA-34a axis. Cancer Science. 2019;**110**(10):3089-3097. DOI: 10.1111/cas.14133

[94] Gomes CP, Nóbrega-Pereira S, Domingues-Silva B, Rebelo K, Alves-Vale C, Marinho SP, et al. An antisense transcript mediates MALAT1 response in human breast cancer. BMC Cancer. 2019;**19**(1):771. DOI: 10.1186/s12885-019-5962-0

Chapter 8

Targeting Axonal Transport: A New Therapeutic Avenue for ALS

Wenting Guo, Laura Fumagalli and Ludo Van Den Bosch

Abstract

Motor neurons have an extreme polarized morphology and heavily rely on efficient cargo transport along axons to maintain their neuronal connections and connections with muscles. Axonal transport deficits have been observed in almost all model systems of ALS. More and more studies have confirmed the close genetic and mechanistic linkage between axonal transport deficits with ALS pathogenesis. Moreover, several therapeutic approaches have been developed to target axonal transport deficits in ALS and showed promising effects in disease models. In this concise chapter, we summarize some major discoveries of axonal transport deficits in ALS pathogenesis and some related therapeutic strategies. We propose that targeting axonal transport may provide a potential therapeutic avenue for ALS.

Keywords: ALS, axonal transport, pathogenesis, therapeutics

1. Introduction

The unique morphological feature of neuronal cells compared with other cell types is their extreme polarity and the incredibly long axons [1]. Although the soma size ranges from 5 μm to 100 μm, axons can be up to 1 m long [1]. Axons keep the efficient communication between soma and axonal terminals [1]. This axonal communication is especially important to motor neuron as they not only need connections with each other but also far reach to muscles in order to control proper muscle contractions [2]. As for ALS, axonal transport defects are one of the most prevalent reported phenotypes from different model systems [2]. In addition, the classical "dying-back" hypothesis could explain the sequence of events during motor neuron degeneration in ALS [3]. The idea is that motor neurons lose their connection with muscle fibers and that the axon retracts back towards the soma, which ultimately results in cell death [3]. This theory is supported by the observation that motor neuron pathology begins at the terminal part of the axon and proceeds in a "dying-back" pattern [3]. In addition, the longest and largest neurites with the highest metabolic demand seem to be the most susceptible to this "dying-back" phenomenon [3].

Mechanistically, axonal transport process relies on three main elements: cargoes, microtubules, and motor proteins and their adaptors [1]. Axonal transport is tracked on microtubules which are polymers of α-tubulin and β-tubulins [1]. Microtubules determine the neuronal polarity with "plus" end at the axonal distal part and "minus" end at the soma part [1]. This polarity allows the directionality of the axonal transport [1]. Kinesin (mainly responsible for anterograde axonal transport, from soma to axonal terminal) and dynein (mainly responsible for retrograde axonal transport, from axonal terminal to soma) are two types of ATP-dependent motor proteins responsible for carrying cargoes along the microtubules [1]. Adaptor proteins are responsible for the connection between motor proteins and cargoes [1]. Axonal transport maintains the efficient supply of cargoes including proteins, RNAs, lipids, and organelles from soma to terminals and is responsible to clear or recycle some misfolded proteins or aggregates under cell stress [1]. It is known that several ALS genes can directly cause axonal transport defects, and axonal transport also actively interacts with other major ALS pathological changes. Gene therapies and compounds that target axonal transport have shown beneficial effects in ALS animal models, and some have already been tested in clinical trials in the context of other diseases. Therefore, a better understanding of transport mechanisms and its role in the disease will open up a new therapeutic avenue for ALS.

2. Axonal transport defects in ALS pathogenesis

2.1 ALS mutations directly interfere with the axonal transport machinery

With the fact that about 10% of ALS cases are considered as "familial ALS" with clear genetic factors involved [4], several ALS gene mutations have been shown which could directly interfere with different aspects of the axonal transport machinery and eventually cause axonal transport defects.

ALS genes that are directly linked to kinesin- and dynein-mediated axonal transport have been uncovered by the discovery of ALS mutations in kinesin family member 5A (KIF5A) and dynactin subunit 1 (DCTN1) [5]. As a member of the kinesin family, KIF5A is mainly expressed in neuronal cells. In the year 2018, two independent large-scale genome-wide association and exome sequencing studies have found that mutations in KIF5A cause ALS [5, 6]. Most of the mutations are loss-of-function mutations that localized in the C-terminal region of the protein where cargoes bind. KIF5A mutations cause altered ATP activity and the dysfunction of kinesin-1 that eventually interfere with the anterograde transport of cargoes along the microtubules [6]. Moreover, for one of the most common ALS-causing genes called fused in sarcoma (FUS) it has been reported that its protein product functions as DNA-/RNA-binding protein that can bind or regulate mRNAs of several other motor proteins including KIF5C, KIF1B, and KIF3A [7], which are actively involved in regulating mitochondrial transport in neurons. Dynactin is a multi-subunit protein that binds and activates dynein by forming a dynein-dynactin motor complex that conveys cargoes in a retrograde transport [8]. The DCTN1 gene encodes dynactin subunit 1, which is responsible for binding microtubules and motor proteins. Heterozygous missense mutations in the DCTN1 gene have been suggested as risk factors for ALS in both sporadic and familial ALS patients [9].

The direct influence from ALS genes to microtubules has been described by the tubulin alpha 4a (TUBA4A) gene and spastic paraplegia 11 (SPG11) gene [10]. Exome-wide variant burden analysis revealed that mutations in TUBA4A associate with both sporadic and familial ALS cases [11, 12]. TUBA4A encodes the tubulin alpha 4A protein. Tubulins are the basic constituents of microtubules [11]. Mutations in TUBA4A destabilize the microtubule network, diminishing its re-polymerization capability that eventually disrupts the transport process [11]. Mutations in the SPG11 gene are the cause of autosomal recessive juvenile-onset ALS. Most of the mutations are loss-of-function mutations [10]. SPG11 encodes a protein called spatacsin, which co-localizes with the cytoskeleton in neurons [13]. Knockdown of SPG11 in mice showed a decreased acetylation level of α-tubulins [13]. With the fact that acetylation of α-tubulin facilitates the stabilization of the microtubules and the binding of motor proteins to the microtubules, silencing SPG11 causes axon outgrowth defects and retrograde axonal retraction in cortical neurons of mice [13]. This is in line with the reduced axon plasticity in human iPSC-derived neurons from patients carrying SPG11 mutations [13]. These studies highlighted the importance of spatacsin in axon maintenance due to insufficient transport and cargo trafficking [13].

Except influencing motor proteins and microtubules, ALS genes can also interfere with axonal transport by affecting the cargoes. As the cargoes can participate into different mechanisms, the interplay between axonal transport and other ALS pathological mechanisms is also linked via cargo-specific transport. Rab proteins are a group of small GTPases that belong to the Ras superfamily [14]. Rabs are responsible for proper vesicle sorting, fission, docking, fusion, and transporting spatially and temporally by switching from an inactive guanosine 5'-diphosphate (GDP)-bound state to an active guanosine 5'-triphosphate [14]. Several Rabs have been reported to play a crucial role in driving neuronal transport in the central nervous system [14]. Mutations in the ALS2 gene cause juvenile-onset ALS. The protein product of the ALS2 gene specifically binds to Rab5 and functions as a guanine nucleotide exchange factor (GEF) for Rab5. The vacuolar protein sorting 9 (VPS9) domain of alsin mediates the activation of Rab5 through endosome and guanine-nucleotide exchanging reaction [14]. Most of the ALS2 mutations are loss-of-function mutations that cause the loss of the VPS9 domain and eventually fail in Rab5 activation [14]. Subsequently, Rab5-dependent endosome and AMPA receptor trafficking are hampered in neuronal culture [15, 16]. The reduction of GluR2-containing AMPA receptors at the synaptic surface in ALS2 knockout neurons results in vulnerability to glutamate toxicity [16]. In addition, more than 20 mutations in the OPTN gene have been described being the causative mutations of ALS [17]. Optineurin, the protein product of OPTN, regulates vesicle trafficking by forming a complex with myosin VI and Rab8 [17]. Myosins are a superfamily of motor proteins that move cargoes along microtubules, while Rab8 is a marker of recycling endosomes. The formation of the complex is Optineurin dependent [17]. This complex localizes at the Golgi apparatus and in cytoplasmic vesicles. It mediates Golgi organization, post-Golgi trafficking, exocytosis, and the basolateral delivery of membrane proteins [17]. In line with this, impaired axonal vesicle transport has been observed in a zebrafish model with optineurin loss. Furthermore, chromosome 9 open reading frame 72 (C9orf72), the most common genetic cause of ALS, is a GEF for Rab8 and is also associated with Rab1 [18, 19]. The knockdown of C9orf72 affects cellular trafficking from the cell membrane to Golgi. Overall, Rab-related transport processes are a good example of the cargo-induced impaired axonal transport in ALS.

2.2 Interplay between axonal transport defects with other ALS pathogenic mechanisms

Based on the genetic discoveries of ALS, intensive studies have proposed several major pathogenic mechanisms that contribute to motor neuron degeneration in ALS. Together with axonal transport defects, other dysfunctional mechanisms such as mitochondrial dysfunction, endoplasmic reticulum (ER) stress, neuroinflammation, excitotoxicity, and abnormal DNA/RNA metabolism have been identified [4]. Although it is still under debate which mechanism plays the vital role in initiating the motor neuron degenerative process, axonal transport defects have been reported to interplay with other mechanisms involved in disease progression.

With the most polarized morphological structure, motor neurons demand high-energy supply to maintain their normal function in controlling muscle contractions [20]. Mitochondria play a pivotal role as the energy supply center in cells. Abnormal mitochondrial morphology and function are observed in postmortem tissues from ALS patients as well as in different ALS animal models [21]. Mitochondrial transport is important to clear the damaged mitochondria and maintain sufficient energy supply from the soma side to the distal side in motor neurons [21]. In line with this, fast motor neurons that have the highest needs of ATP, are more severely affected in ALS compared to slow motor neurons [22]. Therefore, the interplay between mitochondria quality control and transport is crucial for motor neuron survival. Mitochondrial movement along microtubules is controlled by a large complex containing kinesin, dynein, mitochondrial Rho (Miro), and milton [23]. Milton is an adaptor protein that connects Miro and motor proteins. Miro is a GTPase localized to the outer membrane of mitochondria. Miro is regulated by PINK/Parkin, which are genetic modifiers of FUS-induced neurodegeneration [24]. Axonal transport defects have been observed in ALS patient-derived motor neurons and FUS transgenic flies. Decreased expression of either PINK or Parkin is beneficial for reversing the locomotive defects and enhancing the survival of FUS transgenic flies [24]. In addition, overexpression of FUS also increased the ubiquitination of the Miro1 protein [24]. We have observed that mitochondria-associated ER membranes (MAM) are significantly decreased in motor neurons carrying FUS mutation [49]. As Miro1 tends to localize at MAM sites, the decrease of MAM might cause mitochondrial axonal transport reduction due to reduced Miro1-linkage [49]. Similarly, mitochondrial transport defects have also been reported for other ALS genes including vesicle-associated membrane protein-associated protein B/C (VAPB) and C9orf72 genes both in primary cultured neurons and transgenic flies [25]. ALS mutant VAPB interferes with anterograde mitochondrial axonal transport through disrupting Ca^{2+} homeostasis and affecting the amounts of tubulin associated with the Miro1/kinesin-1 complex [25, 26]. The C9orf72 repeat expansion can cause a severe disruption of mitochondrial transport but only a slight inhibition of vesicle transport. Although the exact mechanisms are not clear yet, evidence showed that the toxicity comes from the DPRs translated from the hexanucleotide repeats present in C9orf72 [26].

ER stress is a widely observed pathological change in different ALS models [27]. The ER is responsible for protein synthesis and quality control. Misfolded proteins are one of the earliest finding in models based on SOD1 mutations and later on in other ALS subtypes [27]. In normal conditions, the ER can identify the misfolded protein and trigger the unfolded protein response (UPR) to clear these proteins [27]. While under ER stress, the misfolded proteins will be accumulated without a proper UPR process [27]. It has been suggested that the ER stress can also cause an axonopathy and an irregular microtubule distribution [28]. This has been highlighted by the discovery that mutations in two major genes called PDLA1 and PDLA3 that code ER chaperons are linked with ALS [28]. The ER chaperones or protein disulfide isomerases (PDIs) play a pivotal role in the UPR process [27]. Expression of mutant PDIs in motor neurons affects dendrite outgrowth and causes motor defects in mice [26, 28].

TDP-43 aggregation has been identified as the most prevalent clinical pathological hallmark of ALS patients. In addition, the coding gene TARDBP is an ALS-causing gene. TDP-43 aggregation also widely occurs in other familial as well as sporadic ALS patients. Axonal transport defects have been observed in different model systems of ALS with TDP-43 aggregation [29, 30]. TDP-43 mutations impair mRNA transport in transgenic Drosophila, primary cultured mouse cortical neurons and stem cell-derived motor neurons from ALS patients [29, 30]. Impaired anterograde axonal transport of microtubule plus tip proteins has been observed in primary cultured rat cortical neurons [29]. It has been suggested that cytoplasmic TDP-43 aggregation impairs the cytoskeletal integrity and results in transport deficits [29, 30]. While another study has shown that age-dependent organelle transport defects in iPSC-derived motor neurons from ALS patients carrying TARDBP mutations is independent from TDP-43 aggregation [31], thus, a clear interplay between TDP-43 aggregation and axonal transport still needs to be clarified. Recently, we found that arginine-rich dipeptide repeat proteins (DPRs), which are the pathological translational products from C9orf72 repeat expansion, can cause axonal transport defects in human stem cell-derived motor neurons [32]. We found that several components of the axonal transport machinery interact with arginine-rich DPRs both in vitro and in vivo. It has been proposed that arginine-rich DPRs might directly affect axonal transport through an inhibitory interaction with the microtubule-based transport machinery [32].

DNA damage has been recently proposed as an early pathological change in ALS patients [33]. With the fact that TDP-43 and FUS are DNA-/RNA-binding proteins, the mutations in these genes cause insufficient DNA damage repair and result in motor neuron degeneration [33]. Both DNA damage and distal axonal transport defects have been observed in ALS patients carrying FUS mutations [34, 35]. It has been proposed that DNA damage might play a role in axonal transport defects [34]. When DNA damage is induced in cultured motor neurons, axonal transport defects occur thereafter [34]. In line with this, improving the DNA damage repair process by inhibiting poly(ADP-ribose) glycohydrolase (PARG) shows a rescue of axonal transport defects [34]. Although the exact underling mechanism is not clear yet, it is very likely that DNA damage might induce universal transcriptional changes of some genes that produce proteins that are involved in axonal transport.

3. Therapeutic strategies targeting axonal transport in ALS

As summarized above, different molecular mechanisms underlie axonal transport deficits in ALS. Based on these evidences, therapeutic strategies to restore axonal transport deficits have started to emerge. Given the complexity of the axonal transport machinery and its regulatory mechanisms, multiple approaches have been devised to target the system at different levels.

3.1 Restoring the tracks: approaches to modulate microtubule dynamics

Microtubule-stabilizing agents are currently in clinical use as chemotherapeutic drugs [36]. Compounds that modulate microtubule stability have shown promising results also in the context of neurodegeneration. Epothilone D, for example, has shown beneficial effects in several models of Alzheimer's disease [37, 38]. Because of these findings, Epothilone D underwent a clinical phase 1 trial investigation in patients with mild Alzheimer's disease (NCT01492374, NCT01966666) [39]. Beneficial effects have been reported also for Parkinson's disease [40] and hereditary spastic paraplegia (HSP) [41]. Epothilone D was shown to protect the soma and distal axon of spinal motor neurons early in the disease course of the $SOD1^{G93A}$ model mouse of ALS [42]. However, this was not associated with improved motor performance or survival [42]. While another microtubule-stabilizing agent, Noscapine, was shown to restore axonal transport, to delay the onset of symptoms and to extend the survival of $SOD1^{G93A}$ mice [43].

Pharmacological agents that increase the level of microtubule acetylation have been also used to rescue axonal transport deficits. Acetylated microtubules are considered to be stable, long-lived microtubules [44]. Although the mechanisms and functional consequences of microtubule acetylation is not fully understood [44], it has been suggested that acetylation of α-tubulin promotes the recruitment of molecular motors kinesin-1 and dynein [45, 46], indicating that boosting the level of microtubule acetylation might positively affect intracellular transport. Strong evidence has shown that inhibition of HDAC6, a major tubulin de-acetylating enzyme, stimulates intracellular transport of different cargoes in several models [45–50].

HDAC6 belongs to the histone deacetylases (HDACs) family, and, unlike the other HDACs, HDAC6 is mainly localized in the cytoplasm where it associates with microtubules and with the dynein-dynactin motor complex containing p150glued [51]. In line with these observations, HDAC6 has been implicated in the regulation of cytoskeletal stability, intracellular transport, and cell motility [51, 52]. The beneficial effect of HDAC6 inhibitors has been shown in a broad variety of neurodegenerative diseases. For example, the inhibition of HDAC6 by trichostatin (TSA) increases microtubule acetylation and rescues axonal transport deficit in primary neurons carrying the LRRK2 mutation, which is the most common genetic causes of Parkinson's disease. In addition, in vivo knockdown of HDAC6 and administration of TSA restore locomotor deficits caused by LRRK2 mutation in a Drosophila model [48]. Inhibition of HDAC6 by TSA or Tubastatin A (TubA) restores the levels of acetylated α-tubulin and corrects the axonal transport defects in a mutant HSPB1-induced Charcot-Marie-Tooth disease (CMT) mouse model [47, 53]. TSA also enhances tubulin acetylation and rescues microtubule-based transport deficits observed in Huntington's disease (HD) mutant cells [46]. However, despite the increased microtubule acetylation, the loss of HDAC6 did not rescue neurodegenerative phenotypes and deficits in motor coordination in a HD mouse model [54]. In contrast, genetic deletion of HDAC6 significantly slows disease progression and extends survival of the mutant $SOD1^{G93A}$ mouse model of ALS [55]. The therapeutic potential of HDAC6 inhibition in ALS has been further investigated in FUS iPSC-derived motor neurons [49]. Both TubA and ACY-738 HDAC6 inhibitors rescue the axonal transport deficit in ALS patient-derived motor neurons. This beneficial effect on intracellular transport was further confirmed using HDAC6 antisense oligonucleotides (ASOs) [49]. Furthermore, HDAC6 inhibition increases the acetylation level of α-tubulin in patient-derived motor neurons [49].

Overall, targeting microtubules might represent an interesting therapeutic target in ALS. In particular, modulating the acetylation levels of α-tubulin might be beneficial in restoring axonal transport deficits observed early in the disease course of ALS. HDAC6 inhibitors have shown promising results in the context of ALS; however additional studies are required. For instance, it has been shown that HDAC6 plays an important role in autophagy by promoting the clearance of protein aggregates [56] including mutant SOD1 [57–59]. In this regard, inhibitors of the deacetylation function of HDAC6 that leave the other functions unhampered need to be further validated in the available ALS disease models as they might represent an interesting therapeutic approach.

3.2 Restoring the motors: the role of kinases

Several kinases can directly modulate axonal transport through phosphorylation of motors, adapters, and cargoes [60]. Deregulation of axonal transport by protein kinases has been associated to ALS; therefore the possibility of targeting protein kinases has started to emerge as a novel therapeutic avenue.

An abnormal activation of p38 MAP kinase (MAPK) was reported in mutant SOD1 mice [61–63]. It has been shown that active p38 MAPK phosphorylates kinesin-1, leading to impaired translocation of kinesin-1 along axonal microtubules and inhibition of fast axonal transport [62]. The p38 MAPK inhibitor, SB203580, completely inhibits mutant SOD1-induced apoptosis of motor neurons in vitro [61]. In addition, Semapimod, a p38 MAPK inhibitor potentially suitable for clinical purposes, protects motor neurons from degeneration in vivo, although it only mildly extends the survival of $SOD1^{G93A}$ mice [61]. Importantly, a more recent study has shown that p38 MAPK is directly responsible for $SOD1^{G93A}$-induced axonal transport deficits in motor neurons, further strengthening the link between p38 MAPK and axonal transport [63]. Both genetic and acute pharmacological inhibitions of p38 MAPK rescue axonal transport deficits in motor neurons of $SOD1^{G93A}$ mice both in vivo and in vitro [63]. However, long-term treatment with the p38 MAPKα inhibitor SB239063 (a potentially interesting compound given the ability to cross the blood-brain barrier) has shown significant toxic side effects and, probably because of that, failed to improve axonal transport and muscle function in $SOD1^{G93A}$ mice [63]. Therefore, additional investigation is required to evaluate and optimize the long-term effects of this approach.

Overactivation of GSK3β has been found in the brain and spinal cord of $SOD1^{G93A}$ mice as well as in spinal cord samples from sporadic ALS patients [64–67]. Inhibition of GSK3β was protective in $SOD1^{G93A}$ transgenic mice in some studies [67, 68], but these findings were not confirmed in later ones [69, 70]. Therefore, at present, the involvement of GSK3β in ALS remains controversial. Aberrant activation of cyclin-dependent kinase 5 (CDK5) has been reported in the spinal cord of mouse models of ALS [71–73]. Hyperactivation of CDK5 mis-regulates transport of several cargoes via the Lis1/Ndel1 complex, which directly regulates dynein activity [72]. Reduction of CDK5 activity in neurons from $SOD1^{G93A}$ mice by roscovitine rescues transport deficits [72]. Similarly, inhibition of CDK5 by overexpression of calpastatin improves motor axon survival, delays disease onset, and increases survival of $SOD1^{G93A}$ mice [73].

Overall, modulating kinase activation seems to be beneficial for the transport defects in ALS; however most of these studies focus on the $SOD1^{G93A}$ mouse model. It remains to be determined whether targeting kinases is beneficial also in the context of other ALS-causing mutations. In addition, many protein kinases have multiple targets and are involved in several cellular processes. Therefore a more detailed understanding of kinase signaling pathways is required to effectively implement this strategy.

4. Conclusions and perspectives

Axonal transport defects have been strongly linked with ALS pathogenesis. Different therapeutic strategies have been tested in ALS disease models, showing prospective results. However, a deeper understanding of the pathological mechanisms that are responsible for axonal transport deficit is required to properly target axonal transport in ALS. Most of the therapeutic strategies proposed have been mainly tested in the $SOD1^{G93A}$ transgenic mice, and it is still unknown whether they are beneficial in other familial ALS models. In addition, the use of iPSC-derived motor neurons could potentially help to validate whether these compounds might also be beneficial for the sporadic ALS cases.

Other cellular mechanisms have been shown to be altered in ALS. Therefore it is not easy to clarify whether altered axonal transport causes neuronal degeneration or whether neuronal dysfunction, due to other upstream mechanisms, ultimately leads to malfunctioning of axonal transport. However, the evidence that axonal transport is an early identifiable phenotype in several in vivo models suggests that targeting axonal transport needs to be addressed for an effective treatment.

Relatedly, studies are ongoing to improve the specificity and the ability of drugs to cross the blood–brain barrier. The advent of techniques such as gene therapy and antisense oligonucleotides might speed up the process of effectively targeting axonal transport in patients. The feasibility of gene therapy to ameliorate axonal transport deficits has been already successfully shown in ALS mice [58]. In addition, ASOs that specifically target HDAC6 have been already tested in iPSC-derived motor neurons of FUS patients showing positive effects on transport [49]. Therefore, these approaches might represent an interesting area for future research and might help to identify effective therapeutic strategies.

Author details

Wenting Guo[1,2,3], Laura Fumagalli[1,2] and Ludo Van Den Bosch[1,2]*

1 Department of Neurosciences, Experimental Neurology, and Leuven Brain Institute (LBI), KU Leuven, University of Leuven, Leuven, Belgium

2 Center for Brain & Disease Research, Laboratory of Neurobiology, VIB, Leuven, Belgium

3 Stem Cell Institute (SCIL), KU Leuven, Leuven, Belgium

*Address all correspondence to: ludo.vandenbosch@kuleuven.vib.be

References

[1] Guo W, Stoklund Dittlau K, Van Den Bosch L. Axonal transport defects and neurodegeneration: Molecular mechanisms and therapeutic implications. Seminars in Cell and Developmental Biology. 2020;**99**:133-150. DOI: 10.1016/j.semcdb.2019.07.010

[2] De Vos KJ, Hafezparast M. Neurobiology of axonal transport defects in motor neuron diseases: Opportunities for translational research? Neurobiology of Disease. 2017;**105**:283-299

[3] Dadon-Nachum M, Melamed E, Offen D. The 'dying-back' phenomenon of motor neurons in ALS. Journal of Molecular Neuroscience. 2011;**43**:470-477

[4] Taylor JP, Brown RH, Cleveland DW. Decoding ALS: From genes to mechanism. Nature. 2016;**539**:197-206

[5] Nicolas A et al. Genome-wide analyses identify KIF5A as a novel ALS gene. Neuron. 2018;**97**:1268-1283.e6

[6] Brenner D et al. Hot-spot KIF5A mutations cause familial ALS. Brain. 2018;**141**:688-697

[7] Burk K, Pasterkamp RJ. Disrupted neuronal trafficking in amyotrophic lateral sclerosis. Acta Neuropathologica. 2019;**137**:859-877

[8] Konno T et al. DCTN1-related neurodegeneration: Perry syndrome and beyond. 2017;**41**:14-24. DOI: 10.1016/j.parkreldis.2017.06.004.DCTN1

[9] Münch C et al. Point mutations of the p150 subunit of dynactin (DCTN1) gene ALS. Neurology. 2004;**63**:724-726

[10] Orlacchio A et al. SPATACSIN mutations cause autosomal recessive juvenile amyotrophic lateral sclerosis. Brain. 2010;**133**:591-598. DOI: 10.1093/brain/awp325

[11] Smith BN et al. Exome-wide rare variant analysis identifies TUBA4A mutations associated with familial ALS. Neuron. 2014;**84**:324-331

[12] Perrone F et al. Investigating the role of ALS genes CHCHD10 and TUBA4A in Belgian FTD-ALS spectrum patients. Neurobiology of Aging. 2017;**51**:177.e9-177.e16. DOI: 10.1016/j.neurobiolaging.2016.12.008

[13] Pérez-Branguli F et al. Dysfunction of spatacsin leads to axonal pathology in SPG11-linked hereditary spastic paraplegia. Human Molecular Genetics. 2014;**23**:4859-4874

[14] Mignogna ML, D'Adamo P. Critical importance of RAB proteins for synaptic function. Small GTPases. 2018;**9**:145-157

[15] Lai C et al. Regulation of endosomal motility and degradation by amyotrophic lateral sclerosis 2/alsin. Molecular Brain. 2009;**2**:1-12

[16] Lai C et al. Amyotrophic lateral sclerosis 2-deficiency leads to neuronal degeneration in amyotrophic lateral sclerosis through altered AMPA receptor trafficking. The Journal of Neuroscience. 2006;**26**:11798-11806

[17] Toth RP, Atkin JD. Dysfunction of optineurin in amyotrophic lateral sclerosis and glaucoma. Frontiers in Immunology. 2018;**9**:1017

[18] Song W et al. Mutant huntingtin binds the mitochondrial fission GTPase dynamin-related protein-1 and increases its enzymatic activity. Nature Medicine. 2011;**17**:377-382. DOI: 10.1038/nm.2313

[19] Farg MA et al. C9ORF72, implicated in amytrophic lateral sclerosis and frontotemporal dementia, regulates endosomal trafficking. Human Molecular Genetics. 2014;**23**:3579-3595

[20] Vandoorne T, De Bock K, Van Den Bosch L. Energy metabolism in ALS: An underappreciated opportunity? Acta Neuropathologica. 2018;**135**:489-509

[21] Smith EF, Shaw PJ, De Vos KJ. The role of mitochondria in amyotrophic lateral sclerosis. Neuroscience Letters. 2019;**710**:132933

[22] Le Masson G, Przedborski S, Abbott LF. A computational model of motor neuron degeneration. Neuron. 2014;**83**:975-988

[23] Schwarz TL. Mitochondrial trafficking in neurons. Cold Spring Harbor Perspectives in Medicine. 2013;**5**:pii:a011304. DOI: 10.1101/cshperspect.a011304

[24] Chen Y et al. PINK1 and Parkin are genetic modifiers for FUS-induced neurodegeneration. Human Molecular Genetics. 2016;**25**:5059-5068

[25] Mórotz GM et al. Amyotrophic lateral sclerosis-associated mutant VAPBP56s perturbs calcium homeostasis to disrupt axonal transport of mitochondria. Human Molecular Genetics. 2012;**21**:1979-1988

[26] Baldwin KR, Godena VK, Hewitt VL, Whitworth AJ. Axonal transport defects are a common phenotype in Drosophila models of ALS. Human Molecular Genetics. 2016;**25**:1-15

[27] Jaronen M, Goldsteins G, Koistinaho J. ER stress and unfolded protein response in amyotrophic lateral sclerosis: A controversial role of protein disulphide isomerase. Frontiers in Cellular Neuroscience. 2014;**8**:402. DOI: 10.3389/fncel.2014.00402

[28] Woehlbier U et al. ALS-linked protein disulfide isomerase variants cause motor dysfunction. EMBO Journal. 2016;**35**:845-865. DOI: 10.15252/embj.201592224

[29] Baskaran P, Shaw C, Guthrie S TDP-43 causes neurotoxicity and cytoskeletal dysfunction in primary cortical neurons. PLoS One. 2018;**13**:e0196528. DOI: 10.1371/journal.pone.0196528

[30] Alami NH et al. Axonal transport of TDP-43 mRNA granules is impaired by ALS-causing mutations. Neuron. 2014;**81**:536-543

[31] Kreiter N et al. Age-dependent neurodegeneration and organelle transport deficiencies in mutant TDP43 patient-derived neurons are independent of TDP43 aggregation. Neurobiology of Disease. 2018;**115**:167-181

[32] Fumagalli L et al. C9orf72-derived arginine-containing dipeptide repeats associate with axonal transport machinery and impede microtubule-based motility. bioRxiv. 2019:835082. DOI: 10.1101/835082

[33] Penndorf D, Witte O, Kretz A. DNA plasticity and damage in amyotrophic lateral sclerosis. Neural Regeneration Research. 2018;**13**:173-180

[34] Naumann M et al. Impaired DNA damage response signaling by FUS-NLS mutations leads to neurodegeneration and FUS aggregate formation. Nature Communications. 2018;**9**:335

[35] Wang H et al. Mutant FUS causes DNA ligation defects to inhibit oxidative damage repair in amyotrophic lateral sclerosis. Nature Communications. 2018;**9**:3683

[36] Stanton RA, Gernert KM, Nettles JH, Aneja R. Drugs that target dynamic microtubules: A new molecular perspective. Medicinal Research Reviews. 2011;**31**:443-481. DOI: 10.1002/med.20242

[37] Brunden KR et al. Tau-directed drug discovery for Alzheimer's disease and related tauopathies: A focus on

tau assembly inhibitors. Experimental Neurology. 2010;**223**:304-310

[38] Zhang B et al. The microtubule-stabilizing agent, epothilone D, reduces axonal dysfunction, neurotoxicity, cognitive deficits, and Alzheimer-like pathology in an interventional study with aged Tau transgenic mice. The Journal of Neuroscience. 2012;**32**:3601-3611. DOI: 10.1523/JNEUROSCI.4922-11.2012

[39] Varidaki A, Hong Y, Coffey ET. Repositioning microtubule stabilizing drugs for brain disorders. Frontiers in Cellular Neuroscience. 2018;**12**:226. DOI: 10.3389/fncel.2018.00226

[40] Cartelli D et al. Microtubule alterations occur early in experimental parkinsonism and the microtubule stabilizer Epothilone D is neuroprotective. Scientific Reports. 2013;**3**:1837. DOI: 10.1038/srep01837

[41] Wali G et al. Mechanism of impaired microtubule-dependent peroxisome trafficking and oxidative stress in SPAST-mutated cells from patients with Hereditary Spastic Paraplegia. Scientific Reports. 2016;**6**:27004. DOI: 10.1038/srep27004

[42] Clark JA et al. Epothilone D accelerates disease progression in the SOD1G93A mouse model of amyotrophic lateral sclerosis. Neuropathology and Applied Neurobiology. 2018;**44**:590-605. DOI: 10.1111/nan.12473

[43] Fanara P et al. Stabilization of hyperdynamic microtubules is neuroprotective in amyotrophic lateral sclerosis. The Journal of Biological Chemistry. 2007;**282**:23465-23472. DOI: 10.1074/jbc.M703434200

[44] Janke C, Montagnac G. Causes and consequences of microtubule acetylation. Current Biology. 2017;**27**:R1287-R1292. DOI: 10.1016/j.cub.2017.10.044

[45] Reed NA et al. Microtubule acetylation promotes kinesin-1 binding and transport. Current Biology. 2006;**16**:2166-2172

[46] Dompierre JP et al. Histone deacetylase 6 inhibition compensates for the transport deficit in Huntington's disease by increasing tubulin acetylation. The Journal of Neuroscience. 2007;**27**:3571-3583. DOI: 10.1523/JNEUROSCI.0037-07.2007

[47] d'Ydewalle C et al. HDAC6 inhibitors reverse axonal loss in a mouse model of mutant HSPB1-induced Charcot-Marie-Tooth disease. Nature Medicine. 2011;**17**:968-974

[48] Godena VK et al. Increasing microtubule acetylation rescues axonal transport and locomotor deficits caused by LRRK2 Roc-COR domain mutations. Nature Communications. 2014. DOI: 10.1038/ncomms6245

[49] Guo W et al. HDAC6 inhibition reverses axonal transport defects in motor neurons derived from FUS-ALS patients. Nature Communications. 2017;**8**:861

[50] Govindarajan N et al. Reducing HDAC6 ameliorates cognitive deficits in a mouse model for Alzheimer's disease. EMBO Molecular Medicine. 2013;**5**:52-63. DOI: 10.1002/emmm.201201923

[51] Hubbert C et al. HDAC6 is a microtubule-associated deacetylase. Nature. 2002;**417**:455-458

[52] Valenzuela-Fernández A, Cabrero JR, Serrador JM, Sánchez-Madrid F. HDAC6: A key regulator of cytoskeleton, cell migration and cell–cell interactions. Trends in Cell Biology. 2008;**18**:291-297

[53] Prior R, Van Helleputte L, Benoy V, Van Den Bosch L. Defective axonal transport: A common pathological mechanism in inherited and acquired peripheral neuropathies. Neurobiology of Disease. 2017;**105**:300-320

[54] Bobrowska A, Paganetti P, Matthias P, Bates GP. Hdac6 knock-out increases tubulin acetylation but does not modify disease progression in the R6/2 mouse model of Huntington's disease. PLoS One. 2011. DOI: 10.1371/journal.pone.0020696

[55] Taes I et al. Hdac6 deletion delays disease progression in the SOD1 G93A mouse model of ALS. Human Molecular Genetics. 2013;**22**:1783-1790

[56] Kawaguchi Y et al. The deacetylase HDAC6 regulates aggresome formation and cell viability in response to misfolded protein stress. Cell. 2003;**115**(6):727-738

[57] Lee J-Y et al. Uncoupling of protein aggregation and neurodegeneration in a mouse amyotrophic lateral sclerosis model. Neurodegenerative Diseases. 2015;**15**:339-349

[58] Xie Y et al. Endolysosomal deficits augment mitochondria pathology in spinal motor neurons of asymptomatic fALS mice. Neuron. 2015;**87**:355-370

[59] Gal J et al. HDAC6 regulates mutant SOD1 aggregation through two SMIR motifs and tubulin acetylation. The Journal of Biological Chemistry. 2013;**288**:15035-15045. DOI: 10.1074/jbc.M112.431957

[60] Gibbs KL, Greensmith L, Schiavo G. Regulation of axonal transport by protein kinases. Trends in Biochemical Sciences. 2015;**40**:597-610. DOI: 10.1016/j.tibs.2015.08.003

[61] Dewil M, De La Cruz VF, Van Den Bosch L, Robberecht W. Inhibition of p38 mitogen activated protein kinase activation and mutant SOD1(G93A)-induced motor neuron death. Neurobiology of Disease. 2007;**26**:332-341

[62] Morfini GA et al. Inhibition of fast axonal transport by pathogenic SOD1 involves activation of p38 MAP kinase. PLoS One. 2013;**8**:e65235

[63] Gibbs KL et al. Inhibiting p38 MAPK alpha rescues axonal retrograde transport defects in a mouse model of ALS. Cell Death & Disease. 2018;**9**:596

[64] Hu JH, Chernoff K, Pelech S, Krieger C. Protein kinase and protein phosphatase expression in the central nervous system of G93A mSOD over-expressing mice. Journal of Neurochemistry. 2003;**85**:422-431

[65] Hu JH, Zhang H, Wagey R, Krieger C, Pelech SL. Protein kinase and protein phosphatase expression in amyotrophic lateral sclerosis spinal cord. Journal of Neurochemistry. 2003;**85**:432-442. DOI: 10.1046/j.1471-4159.2003.01670.x

[66] Yang W, Leystra-Lantz C, Strong MJ. Upregulation of GSK3β expression in frontal and temporal cortex in ALS with cognitive impairment (ALSci). Brain Research. 2008;**1196**:131-139. DOI: 10.1016/j.brainres.2007.12.031

[67] Koh SH et al. Role of GSK-3β activity in motor neuronal cell death induced by G93A or A4V mutant hSOD1 gene. The European Journal of Neuroscience. 2005;**22**:301-309. DOI: 10.1111/j.1460-9568.2005.04191.x

[68] Feng H-L et al. Combined lithium and valproate treatment delays disease onset, reduces neurological deficits and prolongs survival in an amyotrophic lateral sclerosis mouse model. Neuroscience. 2008;**155**:567-572

[69] Gill A, Kidd J, Vieira F, Thompson K, Perrin S. No benefit from chronic lithium dosing in a sibling-matched, gender balanced, investigator-blinded trial using a standard mouse model of familial ALS. PLoS One. 2009;**4**:e6489. DOI: 10.1371/journal.pone.0006489

[70] Pizzasegola C et al. Treatment with lithium carbonate does not improve disease progression in two different strains of SOD1 mutant mice. Amyotrophic Lateral Sclerosis. 2009;**10**:221-228. DOI: 10.1080/17482960902803440

[71] Nguyen MD, Larivière RC, Julien JP. Deregulation of Cdk5 in a mouse model of ALS: Toxicity alleviated by perikaryal neurofilament inclusions. Neuron. 2001;**30**:135-147

[72] Klinman E, Holzbaur ELF. Stress-induced CDK5 activation disrupts axonal transport via Lis1/Ndel1/Dynein. Cell Reports. 2015;**12**:462-473

[73] Rao MV, Campbell J, Palaniappan A, Kumar A, Nixon RA. Calpastatin inhibits motor neuron death and increases survival of hSOD1G93A mice. Journal of Neurochemistry. 2016;**137**(2):140-141. DOI: 10.1111/jnc.13536